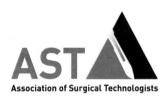

Surgical Technologist Certifying Exam Study Guide
Third Edition

Association of Surgical Technologists
6 West Dry Creek Circle
Littleton, CO 80120
303.694.9130
www.ast.org

ISBN 978-0-926805-66-8

Updated 2015

Fifth printing

III

Table of Contents

IV

Preface

Congratulations! You have chosen to enter the proud profession of surgical technology. The mission statement of AST is to "ensure quality patient care;" in support of the mission AST assists students with meeting their goals to include achieving certification because "every patient deserves a Certified Surgical Technologist."

Historically, AST and its partner organizations, the Accreditation Review Council on Education in Surgical Technology and Surgical Assisting (ARC/STSA) and the National Board of Surgical Technology and Surgical Assisting (NBSTSA) work together to fulfill the commitment to you – the student – at the beginning and end of your educational experience including:

- Supporting the CAAHEP-accredited surgical technology programs to be able to deliver quality education and enable you to pursue a career in the profession.
- Offering continuing education programs and events for surgical technology educators to ensure you are the benefactor of up-to-date instructional methods and techniques.
- Publishing the Core Curriculum for Surgical Technology to establish a uniform standard of knowledge for all graduates of CAAHEP-accredited programs.
- Development of a national certification examination to measure your knowledge through the application of national standards.

This third edition of the AST Surgical Technologist Certifying Exam Study Guide is provided as a review tool to be used in preparing for the national certification examination. Surgical technology educators came together to review every question in order to target the necessary topics to assist you in studying for the examination. Dedicate yourself to passing the examination and join thousands of your colleagues in the OR who already have acknowledged that every patient deserves a Certified Surgical Technologist.

Intro

Preparing for the national surgical technology certification examination offered by the NBSTSA is a challenging task. Preparation started the first day of your program through classroom studies, lab/mock OR and surgical rotation. The goal of this study guide is to serve as a study tool to reinforce the learning that took place while attending the program in preparation to take the certification examination.

The AST Study Guide utilizes information from each major topic provided in the latest edition of the AST Core Curriculum for Surgical Technology as well as the content outline provided in the latest edition of the NBSTSA CST Candidate Handbook. The third edition of the study guide represents a major shift in philosophy, which is applied and presented in a new format. Early in the process of revising the study guide the question was asked, "What do students often do when completing a program?" The answer is obvious – take a lot of tests including preparing to take a national certification examination. Therefore, it only reasoned that the study guide should be presented in such a manner where the student is completing several practice exams as one type of exam preparatory tool.

The Study Guide consists of Section I, "Exam Preparation," that spans chapters one through five and includes: test-taking tips and study strategies, reading techniques, comprehension and retention techniques and methods for studying technical material. Section II is comprised of six practice exams, each of which features 175 multiple choice questions that follow the NBSTSA Examination Content Outline as presented in the CST Candidate Handbook. Practice Exam #6 is provided on the included DVD to give the student an idea of taking the electronic version of the certification examination. A bonus section is provided that is comprised of two basic science practice questions. It is likely that you completed the basic science courses, eg, A&P, Micro, Pharm and Medical Terminology, early in the program. The basic science practice questions are meant to reinforce your review of these subject areas.

The practice exams enable you to measure your understanding of the material by checking your responses with the answers and explanations. Each question is referenced to a specific page in a textbook to facilitate further study. The practice exams are valuable tools that can help you pinpoint the specific subject areas you need to spend more time reviewing, as well as identify your strongest areas that don't demand as much time. Your rate of progress on each practice exam will help establish your study priorities and more efficiently organize your time.

The explanations and textbook references for the practice exam questions are located on the AST website. Placement of this material on the website allows AST the ability to more easily and quickly keep the references up-to-date as new editions of textbooks are published.

Individuals who use this study guide should keep in mind the purposes of the Study Guide and what it can and cannot do.

The Study Guide **will:**
- Provide an overall review of the surgical technology subject areas.
- **Assist** you in identifying the subject areas that you are knowledgeable in and those subject areas that require additional review.
- Provide textbook references that can be used for further study.
- Familiarize you with the format of questions used on the certification examination.
- Provide useful test-taking strategies and review skills.

The Study Guide **will not:**
- Be a repeat of the **comprehensive** education experienced in your class-room.
- Be the single, determining factor for passing the certification examination. The Study Guide should not be relied upon as the only review tool. It is highly recommended that you use a combination of the following of review resources along with the study guide:
    - Review lecture class notes.
    - Review the information in the textbooks that were used during your surgical technology program; in particular review Anatomy & Physiology, Microbiology and Pharmacology since those courses were most likely completed early in the program.
    - Use the NBSTSA Examination Content Outline as a checklist; as each subject area is reviewed check it off.

AST wishes you all the best on taking the certification examination and beginning your career providing quality surgical patient care as a key member of the surgical team!

Acknowledgments

The Association of Surgical Technologists gratefully acknowledges the following individuals for their contributions to the third edition of the Surgical Technologist Certifying Exam Study Guide.

Third Edition of the Surgical Technologist Certifying Exam Study Guide

Study Guide Revision Panel

T Van Bates, CST, BA
Connie Bell, CST, FAST
Angie Burton, CST
Margaret Rodriguez, CST, CSFA, FAST, BS
Roy Zacharias, CST, FAST, BS

Study Guide Reviewers

Theresa Braun, CST
Angie Burton, CST
Ruby Castardo, CST, BSW
Kevin Craycraft, CST, AS-CTE
Suzette Dennington, CST
Audrey Gabel, CST, AAS
Donna Hess, CST
Peggy Howard, RN, BSN, CNOR
Nancy Phelps, CST
Patricia Rich, CST
Kristine Wesse, CST
Jacqueline Woolever, CST

Surgical Instrument Photography

Margaret Rodriguez, CST, CSFA, FAST, BS

AST extends its appreciation to the surgical technology educators who devoted their time to developing and reviewing past editions of the study guide. Their efforts provided a valuable foundation for the publication of the first and second editions.

Second Edition

Connie Bell, CST, FAST
Jeff Bidwell, CST, CSFA, CSA, FAST, MA
Wanda Dantzler, RN, CNOR, CRCST, BSN
Chris Keegan, CST, FAST, MS
Renee Nemitz, CST, RN, BSN
Keith Orloff, CST, FAST
Clifford Smith, RN, CNOR, CRNFA, BSN
Roy Zacharias, CST, FAST, BS

First Edition

Susan Austin, CST
Ruth Ann Briggs, RN, MSN
Dorothy Caracciolo, CST, CSFA
Keith Chase, PhD
Linda Christofi, CST
Diane Fleming, CST
Brenda Frazier, RN, CNOR, BSN, MEd
Julia Halpin, RN, CNOR, MSEd
Chris Keegan, CST, FAST, MS
Rodney Parks, CST
Emily Rogers, CST, FAST, RN, BSN
Margaret Thomas, RN, CNOR, BSN
Ruth Walsh, CST, RN, CNOR, BSN

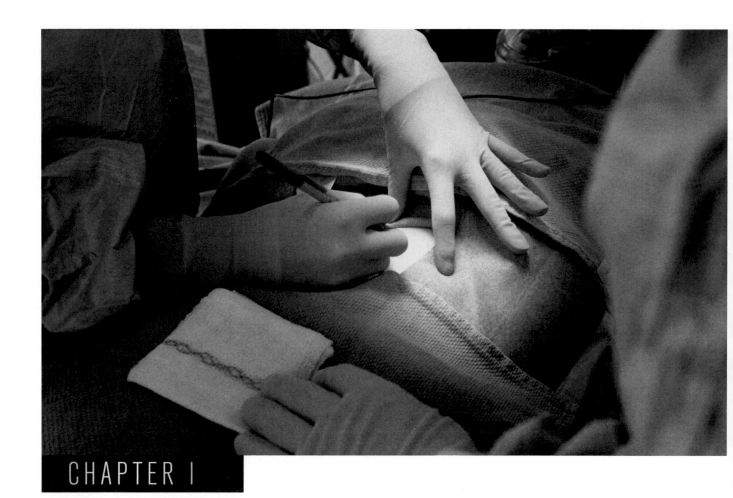

TAKING THE CST EXAM

What is the CST Certification Exam?

Surgical technologists work closely with surgeons, anesthesia providers, registered nurses and other perioperative personnel to provide patient care before, during and after surgery. The contributions of surgical technologists to quality patient care are critical and consequently impose a burden on employers seeking qualified perform at the high standards required individuals who can perform at the high standards required.

Knowledge of asepsis, sterile technique, basic sciences, preoperative, intraoperative and postoperative case management, as well as materials management, sterilization, legal concepts and mastery of specific skills must be evaluated in order to demonstrate a standard of competency.

The certification examination measures on a national scale the broad range of skills and knowledge required by the profession. Receiving a passing score on the certification exam results in the individual earning a public recognition, a credential of certification and placing the CST® designation after their name

Why is Certification Important?

Certification provides evidence of your competence in the related sciences and clinical practice, as well as offering proof of your achievement to employers, colleagues, other health care professionals and the public. The certification credential is confirmation of your professionalism and that's particularly important when working in a field with others who are required to be board certified or licensed, such as surgeons, anesthesia providers, nurses and surgical assistants. Achieving certification proves your commitment to pursue additional education and acquired the basic skills and knowledge of patient care. Even though certification remains voluntary, your efforts illustrate your strength of purpose to your colleagues.

In addition to professional recognition, certification can affect your wages and career opportunities. In a 2003 AST survey, statistics showed that 43% of AST certified members earned at least $14/hour versus only 15% of noncertified members. In the higher compensation ranges, 20% of certified members reported earning $17 per hour versus 5% of noncertified members.

As health care costs including health insurance, is still rising, health care continues to be a challenging area. Without certification you may restricting your future right to practice as more and more states are seeking to enact legislation governing certification. It's possible that your state may not currently require certification, but may do some in the future. And, as more individuals move across state lines to accept a job, you might not be protected to practice if you do not possess certification. Obtaining and staying current on certification ensures that you will be able to practice anywhere at any time.

Who Creates the Certification Exam?

The national certifying examination was first administered in 1970. Four years later, the Liaison Council on Certification (LCC-ST) was established as the certifying agency for surgical technologists. Now known as the National Board of Surgical Technology and Surgical Assisting, the NBSTSA is responsible for establishing the guidelines for certification, as well as preparing, reviewing and establishing the validity of the national certification examination.

The questions and test forms are reviewed by the eight-member CST Examination Review Committee (CST-ERC). The CST-ERC is composed of five practicing CSTs; two surgical technology educators from NBSTSA-recognized programs; and one Board Certified surgeon. The questions are based on the Examination Content Outline developed from the 2012 Job Analysis. The NBSTSA conducts a JA approximately every five years as required by the National Commission for Certifying Agencies (NCCA) for the NBSTSA to maintain accreditation. The JA is a survey that is designed to use detailed specifications to measure what is taking place in a specific professional practice. The input received from CSTs and CSFAs help determine which tasks and skills best represent the specific profession, and therefore, which areas should be addressed in the national certification examination. The content examination outline determines how many questions from a specific area appear on the exam. No two exams are alike, although the questions from each area are the same in each test. The content outline is reviewed consistently to reflect current surgical practices.

The Format of the Certification Exam

The certification examination is a computerized examination composed of 200 multiple-choice questions with four possible answers. There is only one correct answer for each question. Out of the 200 questions, only 175 are scored with 25 pretest items (unscored) randomly distributed throughout the examination for the purpose of analysis and statistical evaluation.

You will have four hours to complete the exam. You may take a break whenever you wish, but you will not be given additional time to make up for time lost during breaks so we advise you to practice pacing yourself. You'll have 240 minutes to take the exam, which breaks down to little more than one minute per question. You may not always need a full minute for each question, but there may be questions that you need to "mark" and return to later. Try to leave time at the end in order to reread any questions that you may have saved or to work through any questions you marked.

> No two exams are alike, although the questions from each area are the same in each test.

The certification examination is broken out by three main divisions: Perioperative Patient Care, Additional Duties and Basic Sciences.

How is the CST Exam Scored?

The 175-item test is scored as a pass/fail examination; you will not receive any numeric score. Before leaving the testing center, you will receive a score report indicating whether you passed.

Individuals who did not pass will receive a report that indicates their efforts were not successful and includes some diagnostic information that will help them determine which areas they need to address and reinforce.

What is a passing score? The NBSTSA states that the minimum number of questions one must answer to pass the national certification examination is 118.

The CST Exam is Predictable

No, we don't have a crystal ball and we can't forecast what exact questions will be on your particular test, but we can offer you some very helpful clues to assist your preparation and guide your review.

Remember, the NBSTSA surveyed practitioners in the 2012 Job Analysis. Their responses about current practice form the basis for questions that are deemed necessary for the field. So, we can look at what areas received focus and project what areas the test will be emphasizing. Of course, no two tests are identical, but they will be constructed using similar percentages of the content areas.

The certification examination organized by three main divisions: Perioperative Patient Care, Additional Duties and Basic Sciences. Each main area is then subdivided into smaller topics.

Topics in Perioperative Patient Care constitute 60% of the certifying examination—that comes out to 105 questions—over half the test! The test examines three central topics of Perioperative Patient Care: Preoperative Preparation, 29 questions; Intraoperative Procedures, 66 questions; and Postoperative Procedures, 10 questions.

Additional Duties constitute 10% of the examination questions and includes Administrative and Personnel, 10 questions; and Equipment Sterilization and Maintenance, 10 questions.

Basic Science questions constitutes 29% of the test and is broken up into the following catergories: Anatomy and Physiology—30 questions; Microbiology—10 questions; and Surgical Pharmacology, 10 questions.

Preparing for the CST Exam

There are several avenues that can assist in prepping for the test. We advise you to employ multiple methods of review so you are thoroughly prepared for the exam.

CHAPTER I
TAKING THE CST EXAM

AST Study Guide

In the AST Study Guide, each exam offers 175 questions to aid your review. Read each question thoroughly and circle the answer. When you have completed the review questions, turn to the answers and explanations; check your work and assign a score. How did you do? For every incorrect answer, read the accompanying explanation.

Be sure to note the areas where you are strong and what topics you need to focus on. This information is critical to determining the most effective use of your study time.

After you have thoroughly reviewed any necessary topics, take the practice test on the DVD included with this study guide. Time yourself and score your test. Did you reach your target? Identify any weak areas and return to your textbooks and old tests to review as needed. Take the test again to see if you can raise your score. Note your time—remember you should leave at least 10 minutes to review your answers.

NBSTSA Candidate Handbook

The Candidate Handbook, published annually by the NBSTSA, is another valuable resource to use for preparing for the exam. The Candidate Handbook provides general information about eligibility, test preparation and exam scheduling.

The exam content outline also is helpful in identifying content areas. It overlaps with information provided within this study guide, but additional review never hurts! Review the material and scrutinize the knowledge area and skills described. Then, take the short 15-question test. Again, how did you do? Identify your strengths and determine what areas need improvement. These questions are similar to the actual examination.

The Candidate Handbook may be downloaded for free on the NBSTSA website, www.nbstsa.org.

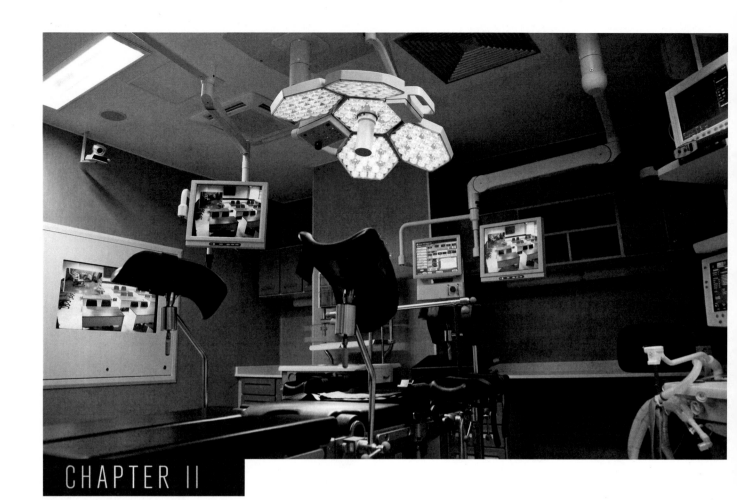

READING
TECHNIQUES

Using Reading Cues

Reading cues can often give clues about the meaning of the material and guide you through the information. The following are types of reading cues that can assist you in determining the correct answer.

- Title and Preface—The words in the title, introductory statements or author's comments can provide you with hints about the selected topic.
- Key Words and Phrases—Important words and phrases are often underlined, boldfaced or italicized and they may appear in different font styles and sizes.
- Action Verbs—Action verbs (ie, cutting, inserting, incising, dissecting, moving) alert you to pay attention to what is happening and why it's happening.
- Key Modifiers—A modifier is a word or phrase that limits or describes another word or phrase (ie, hazard bag or abdominal incision). Quantifiers are a type of modifier and are used as a measurement—how much, how many, how often, etc. Examples include 90 mm Hg, 20% of patients, 12 months, etc.
- Transitions/Relationships—Words such as if, however, since, therefore, then, now, yet, finally, in summation and for example show how ideas are related.
- Listings—Numbers or alphabetic symbols are used to indicate steps, a series of ideas or other sequential arrangements (ie, first, second, third, etc).

Skim and Scan Technique

In skim reading, you read parts of the article quickly to determine whether it is pertinent and should be read in greater detail. This technique is used well for looking for specific facts or ideas. Read the introductory and concluding remarks, check material in italics or boldface type, and if you need a little more information, read the first sentence of each paragraph. If the book is large enough, begin with a topic search in the index.

With scan reading, read only the essentials of an article, noting the high points, to give yourself a general idea of what the material is about, ie, subject, main idea, and the overall way the information is organized. Carefully read the title, introduction and conclusion, including the preface and editorial comments. Note the major divisions of the article. Watch for key statements and reading cues, and review the overall structure of the article.

SUMMARY

- Read title, headers, preface, introductory and concluding paragraphs
- Slow down when you identify reading cues as these indicate important details

- Read the first sentences of each paragraph
- Note the overall structure of the article
- For larger volumes, use the index and table of contents to help find pertinent material

Selecting a Reading Method

Writing styles vary with some concepts more complex and language levels that differ. The reading method or combination of methods you choose need to accommodate the material and the level of comprehension required.

SELECTIVE METHOD—By using the skim and skip technique, you can locate the important information and carefully read through the selected text. This method is preferable for research and reference reading, but is not recommended for general reading, because overall comprehension is minimal.

STRAIGHT-ON METHOD—As implied, you will read every word using this method. The downside to this method is that it tends to be relatively slow and inefficient.

SURVEY METHOD—This method is similar to scan reading as you will look for the overall idea of the general topic, identify key ideas, determine point of view and note high points. This method is good for simple articles and non-narrative material and should not be the main method used when reading detailed or technical material.

FULL COMPREHENSION METHOD—This method encompasses the entire article by mastering the basic and factual details. Reading for full comprehension involves 1) pre-reading by using the scan technique to identify the subject and general theme of the material; 2) reading the article for sequence of ideas, factual details, key terms, cue to limitations and qualification and explanatory remarks; and 3) reviewing and clarifying the material to cement the information in one's mind. Outlining, underlining or summarizing are good tools to use with this process as it can be slow, but thorough. Use this technique for technical reading and for studying.

STRUCTURAL METHOD—You'll identify the structure and overall theme of the article and examine the supporting details in relation to the theme and structure. With this method, you examine the material within the pattern of relationships rather than just reading it. This method is useful when reading textbooks and technical publications or when you need a semi-analytical grasp of the information. Structural analysis and/or underlining should be used with this method.

ANALYTICAL METHOD—As stated, this method analyzes the material presented. Along with using the structural method, this method examines the reader's purpose; the writer's purpose, view, background and status; the selection and relevance of supporting materials; the relevance and relationship to other articles in the same field; and the mode of thinking involved.

This method should be reserved for material of major importance, such as key technical and professional publications at a high level of difficulty and for advanced study purposes.

CRITICAL METHOD—This method relies on your ability and commitment to study as the following items are analyzed and reviewed: the material's implications; validity of thinking used; appropriateness and pertinence of ideas; the validity of the data given; what has been omitted and why; examine possible bias and slanting; and evaluate the conclusions arrived at and their relationship to the data. This method is recommended for reading selected materials of high importance, but also should be used (in a modified form) in ordinary reading.

When studying for a technical exam, the full comprehension method and the structural method will probably be the most useful techniques.

Summary

- Identify your purpose of the reading material in relation to the information provided.
- Determine the level of comprehension you need.
- Pre-read the information to assess the structure, general characteristics and value.
- Consider the time allotted, environment, personal experience and other relevant aspects.

Reviewing

The final review of an article, following the regular reading, is performed for a specific purpose, not merely glancing over the article.

You can strengthen an initially weak reading by reviewing and by scan reading to survey the entire article. Use underlining or notetaking to aid comprehension. For full retention, re-examine the article in the following systematic fashion, and use a moderately rapid scan-reading technique:

1. Re-examine the title, introduction, conclusion, summary, thesis statement, and look for missed reading cues.
2. Scan the entire article quickly, and recheck major divisions and subpoints. Examine the relationship of the key ideas to each other and to the entire article. Check to see if the total organization is evident.
3. Review the relationship of the developmental details and devices to the ideas they support and the type and level of material used.
4. Assemble the results into a summary statement or a fairly complete outline.

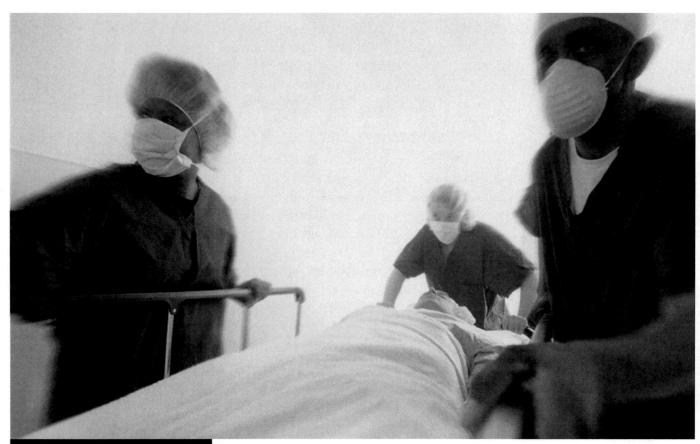

COMPREHENSION AND RETENTION TECHNIQUES

When used together, reading methods and comprehension and retention techniques will help you create a thorough system of study to use when preparing for your upcoming exam.

The following techniques will be covered in this chapter: raising questions, highlighting, taking notes, outlining and summarizing.

Raising Questions

The raising questions technique is useful when combined with skip, skim and scan techniques. As you read quickly through the article, create questions from the article title, headers and key words. The questions should flow naturally from your curiosity about the topic. For instance, "What significance does the key word have in relation to the topic?" Or, "How does one key word relate to a previous key word?"

When you read the text through after raising questions, your mind will automatically begin searching for the answers to the questions you've proposed, aiding your retention. As you find the answers, record them next to your questions so you can later return to them for review and see how much you've retained. When writing out the answers to your questions, include the book title and page number of each answer in case you need to return to the text and review the material in depth.

If there aren't many reader's clues in an article and you find yourself needing more information, form questions that will help identify the details you need. Forming who, what, why, where, when and how questions will help you focus on the answers and the relationship to the material. This is particularly important when studying for an objective exam.

In structural reading, your goal is analytical comprehension, so your questions may consider how the facts are organized, how the parts are interrelated or why the ideas progress in a particular pattern.

Reviewing the questions and written answers is an excellent way to test your retention of the material. If you find a certain question is difficult to answer two or more weeks after studying, review that area of study.

Summary

- Convert the title into a question to discover the main idea
- Scan the article and change the headers and reader cues into questions, using who, what, why, where, when and how
- For greater retention, raise more detailed questions
- Use the appropriate reading method for your level of comprehension, locate answers to the questions you've raised
- Write out the answer to create a short summary of the information

CHAPTER III
COMPREHENSION AND RETENTION TECHNIQUES

Highlighting or Underlining

Highlighting key passages in a text can help you identify and recognize patterns of ideas and facts and their relation to each other.

Highlighting should be used sparingly. Pick out key words and phrases rather than highlighting entire sentences. Pick out only what you need to understand and remember. You should be able to understand the entire article by reading the highlighted words or phrases when finished reading.

Your purpose will also help determine what and how much you highlight.

- If you are reading for facts, underline only those pertinent to your goals.
- For analysis and comprehension, identify how facts and ideas relate by highlighting the key ideas or conclusions along with the facts, indicating their relationships by drawing connective lines or making notes in the margins.

If you are a visual learner, you may want to underline with colored pencils or use different colored highlighters.

Summary

- For comprehension of general information, underline the important points, including subject-significant ideas and few key details
- Underline all major ideas and key factual details for detailed comprehension of scientific and technical articles.
- For analytical comprehension, first underline then outline the material

Taking Notes

Well-written notes save time later by eliminating the need to go back and reread whole chapters or articles. Your desired level of comprehension will determine the amount of detail you include in the notes and should be decided in advance.

When taking notes, use methods that work for you—separate sheets of paper, note cards, a sketch book, etc. Include the subject heading for each section and the source of the note. Recording the source will help you if you need to go back to the original data. Write legibly to simplify the review process.

Procedure for Taking Notes

1. Preread the article and clarify your purpose and the kind of comprehension desired.
2. Decide on the type of notes to use.
3. Read the selection to find pertinent material.
4. Make notes, either during reading or during reviewing.
5. Include only essential data.
6. Review notes immediately to identify any missing details.

To summarize an article, use the scan or skim technique to pinpoint key details and essentail details

Outlining

An outline provides a structural analysis of the text that involves breaking it down into its essential parts for an easier examination of how ideas and facts relate to each other. This technique aids retention by providing a simplified snapshot of the information.

Formal outlines use a sentence or topical approach, and are better for the detailed relationships between ideas and facts. **Informal outlines** may include lists, steps and diagrams, and are useful for visual learners.

The formal outline is where an exact and careful statement of ideas is important, and a sentence outline should be sued. Where such accuracy and completeness of thought is less important, a topic outline can be used. In the latter, the material is reduced to a topic heading complete enough to suggest the essentials of the idea. In formal outline, the sentences of topics should be parallel (similar in style) and should be checked for completeness, clarity of relationships and conformity to the basic structural pattern of the article.

When material is not arranged by specific divisions, a simple type of informal outline may prove more useful. An informal outline is flexible and can be done in margins or on separate pieces of paper. The informal outline can vary based on one's own style and needs. It does not need to parallel the original information, but should still be checked for completeness and clarity.

Formal Outlines

Example–Sentence Outline
Central Idea: Components and functions of the neuron.

I.   Neurons are the basic unit of the nervous system
    A.   This specialized cell communicates with the body through electrical impulses and chemical changes.
    B.   This process of communication coordinates the activities of a human's various systems.
II.   There are three structural classifications of neurons.
    A.   Multipolar neurons are located in the brain and spinal cord.
        1.   Multipolar neurons consist of several dendrites and on axon.
    B.   Bipolar neurons are located in the retina, inner ear and olfactory portion of brain.
        1.   Bipolar neurons consist of one dendrite and one axon.
    C.   Unipolar have only one process and are always sensory.
III.   Neurons are either afferent of efferent.
    A.   Afferent neurons transmit sensory impulses from the receptors back to the brain.

CHAPTER III
COMPREHENSION AND RETENTION TECHNIQUES

B.   Efferent neurons transmit motor impulses from the brain back to receptors.

IV.   Neurons are composed of a cell body, dendrites and the axon.

A.   In addition to parts contained in other cells of the body, neurons contain neurofibrils and Nissl bodies.

1.   Neurofibrils are thread-like structures that provide support for cell processes.

2.   Nissl bodies are membranous sacks that manufacture proteins for cell functioning.

B.   Dendrites are receptive fibers that provide a network for cellular communication.

C.   The cylindrical axon conducts electrical impulses away from the cell body.

1.   The axon can be a single fiber of have many branches (processes) that end in axon terminals.

a.   These processes balloon into synaptic end bulbs that contain sacs called synaptic vesicles.

b.   These vesicles release neurotransmitters into the synapse to influence the actions of other neurons, muscles and glands.

2.   The axon's cytoplasm is surrounded by a plasma membrane called axolemma.

3.   There is no protein synthesis within the axon.

4.   Myelinated axons are produced by Schwann cells or oligodendrocytes.

a.   Axons of the peripheral nerves are surrounded by Schwann cells, whose membranes area made of the lipoprotein myelin.

•   The myelin sheath allows for a faster electrical signal.

•   Outside the myelin sheath is the neurilemma, which contains cytoplasm and nuclei.

b.   The myelinated axons in the brain and spinal cord are produced by oligodendrocytes.

•   Myelinated axons in this area are white, which is the origination of the term white matter in the brain.

Example–Topic Outline

Central Idea: Components and functions of the neuron

    I.   Overview of the neuron
        A.   Basic unit of the nervous system
        B.   Conducts information
        C.   Uses electrical impulses and chemical changes
        D.   Coordinates human activities
   II.   Classifications of neurons
        A.   Multipolar
            1.   Brain and spinal cord
            2.   Several dendrites
            3.   One axon
        B.   Bipolar
            1.   Retina, inner ear and olfactory portion of brain
            2.   One dendrite
            3.   One axon
        C.   Unipolar
            1.   Only one process
            2.   Always sensory
  III.   Functions of neurons
        A.   Afferent
            1.   Sensory
            2.   Transmit from receptors to brain
        B.   Efferent
            1.   Motor
            2.   Transmit from brain to receptors
  IV.   Parts of a neuron
        A.   Cell body
            1.   Same as other cells except …
            2.   Neurofibrils and Nissl bodies
        B.   Dendrites
            1.   Receptive fibers with many branches
            2.   Network for communication
        C.   Axon
            1.   Conducts electrical impulses away from cell
            2.   Axon terminals
                a.   Balloon into synaptic end bulbs
                b.   Contain synaptic vesicles
                    •   Release neurotransmitters into synapse
                    •   Influence neurons, muscles, glands
            3.   Surrounded by axolemma

        4. No protein synthesis
        5. Myelinated axons
            a. Schwann cells
                • Myelin sheath
                • Neurilemma
            b. Oligodendrocyte
                • White matter

Example–Informal Outline

The synapse = small space for neurons to communicate with cells or other neurons

Sender: Axon
    End bulb sacs called synaptic vesicles
Through: Synaptic gap   or   Synaptic cleft
    Via neurotransmitters   via neurotrasmitters
Receiver: Cells   Other axons
    Sodium or potassium ion channels   Receptors differ based on
    Open/close to inhibit/excite   neurotransmitters present

Summarizing

Summarizing is useful for comprehension and retention. All major areas must be covered, including the thesis statement, key ideas and essential supporting details. Deciding what information to select and stripping it down to include the more important material is key to creating an effective summary.

Procedures for Summarizing

- Scan or skim the article, your highlighted text or notes to identify critical parts of the selection
- Select the only significant ideas, key details and essential supporting details
- Summarize from your highlights or notes
- Check the accuracy and completeness of your summary against the original

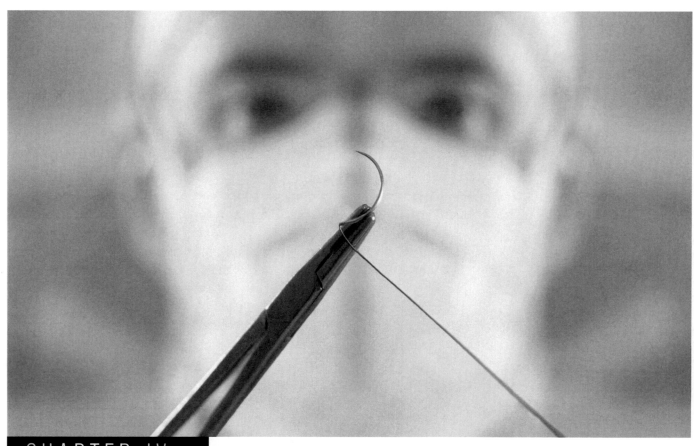

STUDYING
TECHNICAL
MATERIAL

Studying technical material incorporates all the methods and techniques described in previous chapters, but will require serious effort on your part, including focus, concentration and study habits. Some technical information you'll need to understand and some you'll need to memorize.

Concentration is an integral part of the process of studying technical material, but you may find that many elements may add or distract from your ability to concentrate. If you find yourself struggling to concentrate, try these tips.

Purpose: Remind yourself why you're studying. Becoming a Certified Surgical Technologist is important to your career and your future. Your comprehension and retention is critical in your team in the operating room and to your patients.

Interest: If you are struggling to focus on sterile technique or muscular anatomy, stop reading and start over. You may even want to take a quick break to let your mind refresh. Fill up your coffee cup or grab a brain-friendly snack. When you return to your study area, raise questions to help you develop a temporary interest in the information:

- Relate the information to your own experience
- Create a future scenario as a surgical technologist where you would need to know this information

If you still find yourself struggling to stay focused, switch topics and come back to the difficult material at another time.

Study Habits

Creating an environment that is conducive to studying is key. Use these hints when setting up your study environment:

- Select a working spot where you feel comfortable in, but not where you will fall asleep.
- When choosing a place, make sure it is well lit, offers minimal distractions and has plenty of space for you to lay out all your study materials.
- Choose a time that works best for you. Some of us are early birds whereas some of us can't seem to do anything productive until the evening hours. Find the time where your body and mind work best and set a schedule. If you can, make it a habit to study at least a little bit every day at the same place and time.
- Set daily goals, but don't necessarily base them on time. For instance, decide to thoroughly cover one complete chapter instead of studying for two hours. This will help you remind focused on the task at hand instead of the clock.
- Plan breaks accordingly and to give your mind a rest.
- Minimize worries and other personal distractions during your study time.

CHAPTER IV
STUDYING TECHNICAL MATERIAL

- Get adequate sleep each night since people tend to worry or become distracted more easily when they are tired.
- Eat well and exercise. Both elements play a big part for our mind and body to stay healthy and focused.
- Control distractions before they control you. If your stomach is growling, go get something to eat. If your email keeps pinging, close the program while you study. Turn on music only if it helps you concentrate and study with peers or a group only if you benefit from this form of studying.

Memorization Versus Retention

Memorizing plays a big role in this field of practice as you will need to memorize the anatomy and instrumentation involved in each surgery. Thoroughly understanding the basic processes and their underlying rationale is critical.

Memorization Tips

- As you read, take note, mark or list the terms and basic processes that must be memorized.
- Memorizing Latin prefixes and suffixes will make the understanding and memorizing of medical terms easier. The common meaning of prefixes (eg, idio-, neuro-, later-, othr-) and suffixes (-glia, -cele, -oid, -sial) give you instant clues to a word's meaning. Check medical dictionaries for the medical etymology.
- Make flash card of terms and quiz yourself and your classmates.
- Acronyms long have been used in medicine to make technical information easier to remember: MRI—magnetic resonance imaging; ANS—autonomic nervous system; etc. Form your own acronyms to help yourself remember small sets of material.
- Create mnemonic phrases and sentences to help memorize groups of information.

  Here are examples of sentences surgical technology students have used to memorize the cranial nerves—olfactory, optic, oculomotor, trochlear, trigeminal, abducens, facial, vestibulocochlear, glossopharyngeal, vagus, accessory, hypoglossal:

  1. *Old Opie Occasionally Tries Trigonometry And Feels Very Gloomy, Vague, and Hypoactive*
  2. *On Old Olympus Towering Top, A Fair Voluptuous German Vaults and Hops*
- Memorize material together that will be recalled together. Learning the 12 cranial nerves in two parts, for instance, would be more difficult than learning and recalling them together.

- Visual learners should create vivid, colorful images, diagrams or flow charts. Create word pictures of terms. For example, to recall which is the Kittner sponge, imagine a kitten batting the tiny roll of cotton across the operating room floor.
- Auditory learners should try to teach the material to someone else. Thinking through the explanation and hearing yourself explain it will help you memorize it.
- Auditory learners can also pay attention to patterns of inflection in a series of words. Poetry and music rely on rhythm and inflection, and are easier to remember. Try adding a tune to the words you need to memorize.
- Practice recalling information by bringing to mind what you've memorized while doing something completely different, such as waiting in the line at the grocery store. Recalling the material out of context of a surgical or educational setting will help you access it during the testing environment.
- Take the time to thoroughly understand what you're trying to retain. Look up any vague aspects.
- Review old tests. Go back to the original sources to find correct answers to the questions you missed.
- REVIEW THE MATERIAL. Again, and again, and again, and again ... you get the point! Repetition is the key.

CHAPTER IV
STUDYING TECHNICAL MATERIAL

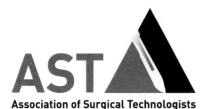
Directions: *Be sure to read each question carefully and select the best answer. You have four hours to complete the test. After finishing the test, review the answers and score your exam.*

In order to pass the CST examination, you must answer 118 questions correctly. If you achieved that score—congratulations! If not, take the time to identify what topics you struggled with and review the appropriate material.

1. **Which of the following structures is located in the alveolar processes?**

    o A. Teeth
    o B. Villi
    o C. Sinuses
    o D. Tonsils

2. **Which of the following is the wound classification for a bronchoscopy?**

    o A. Clean
    o B. Contaminated
    o C. Dirty and infected
    o D. Clean-contaminated

3. **The enzyme used to soften the zonules of the lens before cataract surgery is:**

    o A. Atropine sulfate
    o B. Alpha-chymotrypsin
    o C. Acetylcholine chloride
    o D. Pilocarpine hydrochloride

4. **How should the stretcher be oriented when necessary to use an elevator to transport a patient to the OR?**

    o A. Place stretcher sideways in elevator
    o B. Enter head first, exit feet first
    o C. Position in elevator is irrelevant
    o D. Enter feet first, exit head first

5. **Which of the following is a curved, transverse incision across the lower abdomen frequently used in gynecological surgery?**

    o A. Midline
    o B. Paramedian
    o C. McBurney's
    o D. Pfannenstiel

6. **When perforated metal trays are placed on the shelves of the steam sterilizing cart, they should be positioned:**

   o A. Flat

   o B. Upside down

   o C. Vertical

   o D. Angled

7. **Hyperkalemia is a high concentration of:**

   o A. Calcium

   o B. Nitrogen

   o C. Potassium

   o D. Albumin

8. **Which of the following tissues are cut using curved Mayo scissors?**

   o A. Fascia

   o B. Periosteum

   o C. Dura mater

   o D. Arterial wall

9. **Which laser beam can travel through clear tissues without heating them?**

   o A. Argon

   o B. Excimer

   o C. Carbon dioxide

   o D. Neodymium: YAG

10. **Permission for treatment given with full knowledge of the risks is a/an:**

    o A. Tort

    o B. Malpractice

    o C. Personal liability

    o D. Informed consent

11. **Which portion of the stomach surrounds the lower esophageal sphincter?**

    o A. Cardia

    o B. Fundus

    o C. Pylorus

    o D. Antrum

12. **Low level disinfectants kill most microbes, but do not destroy:**

    o A. Viruses

    o B. Bacteria

    o C. Fungi

    o D. Spores

13. **Syndactyly refers to:**

o A. Cleft palate

o B. Webbed fingers

o C. Fused tarsals

o D. Torn ligaments

14. **The surgical pack utilized to create the sterile field should be opened on the:**

o A. Stretcher

o B. OR table

o C. Backtable

o D. Mayo stand

15. **The islets of Langerhans secrete:**

o A. Bile

o B. Insulin

o C. Intrinsic factor

o D. Inhibiting hormones

16. **What type of procedure would involve the removal of teeth?**

o A. Cleft palate repair

o B. Arch bar application

o C. Extractions

o D. Implants

17. **Which organism is a normal resident flora of the intestinal tract?**

o A. *Escherichia coli*

o B. *Staphylococcus aureus*

o C. *Pseudomonas aeruginosa*

o D. *Clostridium tetani*

18. **Where should the first scrub surgical technologist stand when handing towels to the surgeon to square off an incision site?**

o A. Opposite side from surgeon

o B. Same side as surgeon

o C. Foot of OR table

o D. Head of OR table

19. **A properly performed surgical scrub renders the skin:**

o A. Sterile

o B. Disinfected

o C. Surgically clean

o D. Moistened and dehydrated

20. Through which of the following do the common bile duct and the pancreatic duct empty?

    o A. Ampulla of Vater

    o B. Duct of Santorini

    o C. Wirsung's duct

    o D. Sphincter of Oddi

21. Which of the following identifiers must be verified by the patient or their ID bracelet prior to transporting a patient to the OR?

    o A. Name, social security #, physician

    o B. Name, medical record #, allergies

    o C. Name, date of birth, diagnosis

    o D. Name, date of birth, physician

22. What are spiral-shaped bacteria called?

    o A. Cocci

    o B. Bacilli

    o C. Spirilli

    o D. Diplococci

23. The primary function of the gallbladder is to:

    o A. Store bile

    o B. Produce bile

    o C. Emulsify fats

    o D. Metabolize fats

24. Which of the following is a non-sterile member of the surgical team?

    o A. Surgeon

    o B. Circulator

    o C. Surgical assistant

    o D. Surgical technologist

25. Which of the following is not a benefit of using surface-mounted sliding doors for access to the operating room?

    o A. Uses less space for opening

    o B. Aid in controlling temperature

    o C. Eliminate air turbulence

    o D. Provides for thorough cleaning

26. What are the three factors for reducing ionizing radiation exposure?

    o A. Type of procedure, equipment, radiation dose

    o B. Exposure, frequency, concentration

    o C. Time, shielding, distance

    o D. Site, age, gender

27. **Which is the first part of the small intestine?**

o A. Duodenum

o B. Jejunum

o C. Ileum

o D. Cecum

28. **What is the surgical position frequently used for patients undergoing kidney surgery?**

o A. Prone

o B. Lateral

o C. Supine

o D. Lithotomy

29. **How are rickettsiae transmitted?**

o A. Arthropod bites

o B. Physical contact

o C. Blood exposure

o D. Airborne organisms

30. **Which of the following is an examination of the cervix using a binocular microscope?**

o A. Colposcopy

o B. Laparoscopy

o C. Urethroscopy

o D. Hysteroscopy

31. **Compression of the heart from excessive fluid or blood buildup is called:**

o A. Tamponade

o B. Pericarditis

o C. Infarction

o D. Cardiomyopathy

32. **Which surgical team member determines when the patient can be transported from the OR to the PACU?**

o A. Anesthesia provider

o B. Circulator

o C. Surgeon

o D. Surgical technologist

33. **Which suffix means surgical puncture to remove fluid?**

o A. –dynia

o B. –tomy

o C. –lysis

o D. –centesis

34. **To which portion of the colon is the appendix attached?**

o   A.   Ascending

o   B.   Descending

o   C.   Cecum

o   D.   Sigmoid

35. **Which laboratory test determines bacterial identification?**

o   A.   Gram stain

o   B.   Manual count

o   C.   Prothrombin time

o   D.   Gel electrophoresis

36. **Medication used to dilate the pupil is called:**

o   A.   Miotics

o   B.   Myopics

o   C.   Mydriatics

o   D.   Muscarinics

37. **Which of the following drapes is non-fenestrated?**

o   A.   Laparotomy

o   B.   U-drape

o   C.   Transverse

o   D.   Craniotomy

38. **Under what circumstances would it be appropriate to remove a patient's identification bracelet?**

o   A.   During insertion of an IV catheter

o   B.   Never until patient is discharged from facility

o   C.   Postoperatively when taken to the nursing unit

o   D.   When patient is awake and alert and can verbally identify self

39. **What is the position most commonly used for mitral valve replacement?**

o   A.   Prone

o   B.   Sims

o   C.   Supine

o   D.   Kraske

40. **Which laser is best used during a vitrectomy?**

o   A.   Carbon dioxide

o   B.   Nd:YAG

o   C.   Excimer

o   D.   Argon

41. **Which of the following monitors provides positive assurance of sterility?**

  o A. Clerical
  o B. Mechanical
  o C. Biological
  o D. Chemical

42. **The apron-like structure attached to the greater curvature of the stomach is the:**

  o A. Omentum
  o B. Mesentery
  o C. Ligamentum
  o D. Peritoneum

43. **Which microbes live without oxygen?**

  o A. Aerobes
  o B. Anaerobes
  o C. Capnophiles
  o D. Microaerophiles

44. **Which of the following is an abnormal tract between two epithelium-lined surfaces that is open at both ends?**

  o A. Epithelialization
  o B. Fistula
  o C. Herniation
  o D. Sinus

45. **What is the action of antagonist drugs?**

  o A. Inhibit the clotting process
  o B. Achieve neuroleptanesthesia
  o C. Increase the effects of opiates
  o D. Counteract the action of another drug

46. **Which of the following directional terms describes the type of skin prep of an entire extremity?**

  o A. Spiral
  o B. Horizontal
  o C. Longitudinal
  o D. Circumferential

47. **What organs are excised if an ovarian tumor is malignant?**

  o A. Bilateral ovaries only
  o B. Bilateral fallopian tubes and ovaries, uterus
  o C. Unilateral involved ovary and fallopian tube
  o D. Unilateral involved ovary and fallopian tube, uterus

48. **Which term refers to an abnormal thoracic curve of the spine referred to as "hunchback"?**

- o A. Lordosis
- o B. Scoliosis
- o C. Kyphosis
- o D. Alkalosis

49. **What is the medical term for a bunion?**

- o A. Talipes valgus
- o B. Hallux valgus
- o C. Hallux varus
- o D. Talipes varus

50. **What incision is also known as a lower oblique?**

- o A. Inguinal
- o B. Paramedian
- o C. Infraumbilical
- o D. Thoracoabdominal

51. **The small intestine attaches to the posterior abdominal wall by the:**

- o A. Mesentery
- o B. Peritoneum
- o C. Falciform ligament
- o D. Lesser omentum

52. **What is the term for a relationship in which two organisms occupy the same area and one organism benefits while the other is unharmed?**

- o A. Commensalism
- o B. Neutralism
- o C. Mutualism
- o D. Parasitism

53. **A topical steroid used to reduce inflammation after eye surgery is:**

- o A. Depo-Medrol
- o B. Miochol
- o C. Healon
- o D. Wydase

54. **How is the surgical informed consent signed if an adult patient is illiterate?**

- o A. Authorized individual signs patient's name
- o B. Patient marks with an "X" and witness verifies
- o C. RN and surgeon sign that patient gave consent
- o D. Surgeon and Risk Manager sign consent

55. **What direction should the stretcher be oriented when transporting a patient to the OR department?**

   o A. Feet first, side rails up
   o B. Feet first, side rails down
   o C. Head first, side rails up
   o D. Head first, side rails down

56. **Which of the following routine preoperative laboratory studies would be ordered for premenopausal women with no history of hysterectomy?**

   o A. HCG
   o B. HBV
   o C. HIV
   o D. HDL

57. **Which portion of the surgical gown is considered non-sterile?**

   o A. Outside closure ties
   o B. Two inches below neckline to table level
   o C. Upper arms, neckline and axillary region
   o D. Sleeves; two inches above the elbows to the cuffs

58. **What is the name of the urinary catheter with a small, curved tapered tip used on patients with urethral strictures?**

   o A. Iglesias
   o B. Coude
   o C. Pigtail
   o D. Bonanno

59. **What is the surgical position commonly used for thyroid and gallbladder surgery?**

   o A. Supine
   o B. Fowler's
   o C. Reverse Trendelenburg
   o D. Lateral Kidney

60. **A congenital defect in which the fetal blood vessel between the pulmonary artery and aorta does not close is:**

   o A. Coarctation of the aorta
   o B. Patent ductus arteriosus
   o C. Tetralogy of Fallot
   o D. Ventricular septal defect

61. **Which of the following is a commonly used preservative for tissue specimens?**

   o A. Saline
   o B. Formalin
   o C. Ethyl alcohol
   o D. Lugol's solution

62. **What is the first step taken for an initial incorrect closing sponge count?**

o A. Notify surgeon and repeat count

o B. X-ray patient

o C. Check body cavity

o D. Complete incident report

63. **The mumps may be diagnosed by finding inflammation in which of the following glands?**

o A. Sublingual

o B. Thyroid

o C. Parotid

o D. Submandibular

64. **What institutional document is completed when an adverse or unusual event takes place in the OR that may have legal consequences for the staff or patient?**

o A. Incident report

o B. Operative record

o C. Deposition report

o D. Advance directive

65. **For which procedure would Trendelenburg position provide optimal visualization?**

o A. Cholecystectomy

o B. Hysterectomy

o C. Thyroidectomy

o D. Acromioplasty

66. **Which of the following is a nonadherent dressing?**

o A. Kling

o B. Adaptic

o C. Collodion

o D. Elastoplast

67. **Which of the following is a fenestrated drape?**

o A. Incise

o B. U-drape

o C. Aperture

o D. Half-sheet

68. **Which of the following terms describes a hernia that occurs within Hesselbach's triangle?**

o A. Direct

o B. Indirect

o C. Femoral

o D. Hiatal

69. **Which of the following incisions is oblique?**

o A. Epigastric
o B. Kocher
o C. Paramedian
o D. Pfannenstiel

70. **Which of the following dilators are used in the common duct?**

o A. Pratt
o B. Van Buren
o C. Bakes
o D. Hegar

71. **Which of the following is a mechanical method of hemostasis?**

o A. Laser
o B. Ligature
o C. Thrombin
o D. Electrosurgery

72. **The organ that is connected by a duct to the duodenum is the:**

o A. Pancreas
o B. Gallbladder
o C. Stomach
o D. Liver

73. **A brain tumor causing alteration of muscle tone, voluntary muscle coordination, gait and balance would likely be located in the:**

o A. Diencephalon
o B. Cerebellum
o C. Medulla
o D. Pons

74. **What is the term for a relationship that benefits one organism at the expense of another?**

o A. Commensalism
o B. Neutralism
o C. Mutualism
o D. Parasitism

75. **What type of disease is characterized by rapid onset and a rapid recovery?**

o A. Acute
o B. Chronic
o C. Primary
o D. Asymptomatic

76. **Which organelle is responsible for the production of energy?**

o A. Lysosomes

o B. Mitochondria

o C. Golgi complex

o D. Endoplasmic reticulum

77. **What type of anesthesia is a combination of inhalation and intravenous drugs?**

o A. Spinal

o B. Sedation

o C. Regional

o D. Balanced

78. **Who is ultimately responsible for obtaining the surgical informed consent?**

o A. Guardian

o B. Patient

o C. Surgeon

o D. Nurse

79. **What position is most commonly used for neurosurgical procedures?**

o A. Supine

o B. Semi-Fowler's

o C. Trendelenburg

o D. Lithotomy

80. **The outer layer of the intestine is the:**

o A. Mucosa

o B. Serosa

o C. Muscularis

o D. Submucosa

81. **Which of the following solutions should be used to prep the donor site for a split-thickness skin graft?**

o A. Iodophor

o B. Avagard®

o C. Chlorhexidine

o D. Merthiolate

82. **What type of drape would be used for a flank procedure?**

o A. Transverse

o B. Extremity

o C. Aperture

o D. Perineal

83. **Where should the safety strap be placed on a patient who is in the supine position?**

o A. Below the knees

o B. Across the waist

o C. Over the thighs

o D. Across the abdomen

84. **Which surgical procedure is performed to correct an abnormality in which the urethral meatus is situated on the superior aspect of the penis?**

o A. Hypospadias repair

o B. Epispadias repair

o C. Meatotomy

o D. Ureteroneocystostomy

85. **Which thermal method of hemostasis utilizes intense, focused light?**

o A. Laser

o B. Bipolar

o C. Harmonic

o D. Monopolar

86. **What is the most common cause of intracerebral hemorrhage?**

o A. Hypotension

o B. Hypertension

o C. Meningioma

o D. Meningitis

87. **The larynx is located between the:**

o A. Pharynx and trachea

o B. Nasal cavity and pharynx

o C. Trachea and bronchi

o D. Nasal and oral cavities

88. **The most common cause of retinal detachment is:**

o A. Aging

o B. Trauma

o C. Glaucoma

o D. Inflammation

89. **What postoperative complication is associated with total hip arthroplasty?**

o A. Compartment syndrome

o B. Upper extremity weakness

o C. Urinary incontinence

o D. Pulmonary embolism

90. **Which of the following is a type of passive drain?**

o A. Penrose

o B. Hemovac

o C. Pleur-evac

o D. Jackson-Pratt

91. **The vocal cords are located in the:**

o A. Pharynx

o B. Larynx

o C. Trachea

o D. Bronchus

92. **What type of acquired immunity is a vaccination?**

o A. Artificial passive

o B. Artificial active

o C. Natural passive

o D. Natural active

93. **When would the anesthesia provider request cricoid pressure?**

o A. Bier block

o B. Epidural injection

o C. Endotracheal intubation

o D. Endotracheal extubation

94. **Which instrument would be used during a keratoplasty to remove the cornea?**

o A. Trephine

o B. Westcott

o C. Oculotome

o D. Phacoemulsifier

95. **What is the required minimum number of individuals to transfer an incapacitated patient from the OR table to the stretcher?**

o A. 3

o B. 4

o C. 5

o D. 6

96. **Which of the following regulations states that blood and body fluids should be considered infectious?**

o A. Body Substance Isolation Rules

o B. Medical Device Safety Act

o C. Postexposure Prophylaxis

o D. Standard Precautions

97. **Which of the following is a major source of distress for toddler and preschool age patients being transported to the operating room?**

   o A.   Room temperature change
   o B.   Lack of communication
   o C.   Fear of anesthesia
   o D.   Separation anxiety

98. **Which structure has oral, nasal, and laryngeal divisions?**

   o A.   Esophagus
   o B.   Trachea
   o C.   Pharynx
   o D.   Glottis

99. **Otoplasty is performed to correct a congenital deformity of which structure?**

   o A.   Mouth
   o B.   Nose
   o C.   Ear
   o D.   Eye

100. **An injury a patient sustains as a result of the care given by a healthcare professional is called:**

   o A.   Iatrogenic
   o B.   Liability
   o C.   Battery
   o D.   Tort

101. **The highly vascular layer of the eye that absorbs light rays and nourishes the retina is the:**

   o A.   Sclera
   o B.   Iris
   o C.   Choroid
   o D.   Macula

102. **According to Maslow's hierarchy of needs, which of the following is the patient satisfying when he/she trusts the surgical team's abilities?**

   o A.   Physiological
   o B.   Belonging
   o C.   Esteem
   o D.   Safety

103. **Which aneurysm usually develops between the renal and iliac arteries?**

   o A.   Ascending thoracic
   o B.   Aortic arch
   o C.   Descending thoracic
   o D.   Abdominal aortic

104. **The agent used to flush an artery to prevent clotting is:**

o A. Heparin

o B. Thrombin

o C. Protamine sulfate

o D. Ringer's lactate

105. **What is the next step for reattachment of a severed digit after debridement?**

o A. Vessel reanastomosis

o B. Nerve reanastomosis

o C. Bone-to-bone fixation

o D. Tendon-to-tendon fixation

106. **What type of skin graft includes the epidermis and all of the dermis?**

o A. Composite

o B. Split-thickness

o C. Pedicle

o D. Full-thickness

107. **Which muscle type is striated and voluntary?**

o A. Visceral

o B. Heart

o C. Skeletal

o D. Cardiac

108. **Which of the following terms refers to absence of the external ear?**

o A. Microtia

o B. Anophthalmia

o C. Cheiloschisis

o D. Ectrosyndactyly

109. **What is the recommended maximum time limit for a tourniquet to remain inflated on an adult lower extremity?**

o A. 30 minutes

o B. 60 minutes

o C. 1 ½ hours

o D. 2 ½ hours

110. **Which organism causes gas gangrene?**

o A. *Clostridium perfringens*

o B. *Clostridium botulinum*

o C. *Staphylococcus aureus*

o D. *Staphylococcus epidermidis*

111. **Chest rolls should span the distance bilaterally between which two anatomical structures?**

o A. Nipple to umbilicus

o B. Iliac crest to iliac crest

o C. Scapula to gluteus maximus

o D. Acromioclavicular joint to iliac crest

112. **Which ossicle of the middle ear covers the oval window?**

o A. Malleus

o B. Incus

o C. Stapes

o D. Utricle

113. **What is another name for the Kraske position?**

o A. Dorsal recumbent

o B. Jackknife

o C. Trendelenburg

o D. Beach chair

114. **What type of sponge is tightly rolled cotton tape used by surgeons for blunt dissection?**

o A. Raytec

o B. Kittner

o C. Weck-Cel

o D. Cottonoid

115. **Which of these instruments would be used during a keratoplasty?**

o A. Kilner hook

o B. Bowman probe

o C. Kerrison rongeur

o D. Cottingham punch

116. **A partially dislocated joint is called:**

o A. Subluxation

o B. Malrotation

o C. Avulsion

o D. Malunion

117. **What condition is characterized by build-up of fatty deposits such as cholesterol?**

o A. Embolism

o B. Thrombosis

o C. Arteriospasm

o D. Atherosclerosis

118. **Plaster rolls for casting should be submerged in which of the following?**

o A. Lukewarm saline

o B. Lukewarm water

o C. Cold saline

o D. Cold water

119. **The avascular, clear portion of the eye covering the iris is the:**

o A. Cornea

o B. Sclera

o C. Pupil

o D. Conjunctiva

120. **How often should surgical masks be changed?**

o A. After lunch

o B. Twice-a-day

o C. After each case

o D. Every two hours

121. **Which term describes a rod-shaped microorganism?**

o A. Coccus

o B. Bacillus

o C. Spirillum

o D. Helical

122. **When using the warm cycle of the EtO sterilizer, what is the minimum sterilization temperature in Fahrenheit?**

o A. 55

o B. 65

o C. 75

o D. 85

123. **Which of the following actions would be a violation of aseptic technique?**

o A. Cuffing the hands within the drape

o B. Sterile person reaching over sterile surface

o C. Repositioning penetrating towel clip

o D. Sterile surgical members passing face-to-face

124. **Which legal principle applies when the patient is given the wrong dose of the local anesthetic?**

o A. Res ipsa loquitor

o B. Respondeat superior

o C. Bona fide

o D. Assault

125. **The space between the vocal cords is called the:**

   o A. Epiglottis
   o B. Glottis
   o C. Vocal fold
   o D. Cricoid cartilage

126. **Which bacteria could be found in a penetrating wound caused by a rusty nail?**

   o A. *Treponema pallidum*
   o B. *Bacillus anthracis*
   o C. *Clostridium tetani*
   o D. *Helicobacter pylori*

127. **Which of the following retractors is used for spinal nerve roots?**

   o A. Taylor
   o B. Love
   o C. Cushing
   o D. Meyerding

128. **What is another name for the electrosurgical unit's patient return electrode?**

   o A. Cautery
   o B. Generator
   o C. Foot pedal
   o D. Grounding pad

129. **What size of Foley catheter is commonly used for adults?**

   o A. 8 Fr
   o B. 12 Fr
   o C. 16 Fr
   o D. 24 Fr

130. **Which of the following tumors is typically benign, encapsulated, and arises from tissue covering the central nervous system structures?**

   o A. Meningioma
   o B. Astrocytoma
   o C. Schwannoma
   o D. Oligodendroglioma

131. **The fibrous white layer that gives the eye its shape is the:**

   o A. Iris
   o B. Cornea
   o C. Sclera
   o D. Choroid

132. **What is the term for thread-like appendages that provide bacteria with motion?**

o A. Flagella

o B. Fimbriae

o C. Mesosomes

o D. Mitochondria

133. **What surgical position provides optimal visualization of the lower abdomen or pelvis?**

o A. Fowler's

o B. Reverse Trendelenburg

o C. Trendelenburg

o D. Kraske

134. **How many hours must an item submerse in glutaraldehyde to sterilize?**

o A. 7

o B. 8

o C. 9

o D. 10

135. **When a patient's blood pressure is 135/81, 135 refers to:**

o A. Diastolic

o B. Systolic

o C. Pedal pulse

o D. Apical pressure

136. **A term referring to a waxy secretion in the external ear canal is:**

o A. Mucous

o B. Sputum

o C. Cerumen

o D. Perilymph

137. **Which of the following is an ossicle of the middle ear?**

o A. Pinna

o B. Incus

o C. Labyrinth

o D. Vestibule

138. **What is the term for the process of removing blood from an extremity prior to inflating the pneumatic tourniquet?**

o A. Exsanguination

o B. Extravasation

o C. Evisceration

o D. Evacuation

139. **Which of the following may require probing and dilating in pediatric patients with upper respiratory infections?**

   o A. Sinus cavities
   o B. Eustachian tube
   o C. Nasolacrimal duct
   o D. Tympanic membrane

140. **Which surgical team member is responsible for setting up the sterile field?**

   o A. Surgical first assistant
   o B. Surgical technologist
   o C. Circulating nurse
   o D. Surgeon

141. **In what circumstances would cell-saver transfusion be contraindicated?**

   o A. Anemic patients
   o B. Diabetic patients
   o C. Cancer procedures
   o D. Orthopedic procedures

142. **Use of an intraluminal (circular) stapler (EEA) would be indicated for which of the following surgical procedures?**

   o A. Pancreatectomy
   o B. Cholecystectomy
   o C. Polypectomy
   o D. Sigmoidectomy

143. **Satinsky, Herrick, and Mayo clamps may be specifically used on which of the following structures?**

   o A. Kidney pedicle
   o B. Seminal vesicle
   o C. Bladder neck
   o D. Prostate gland

144. **The nasal cavity is divided into two portions by the:**

   o A. Ethmoid
   o B. Septum
   o C. Vomer
   o D. Sphenoid

145. **Which of the following is used by the surgeon to intermittently remove prostatic tissue fragments during a TURP?**

   o A. Randall forceps
   o B. Wire snare
   o C. Ellik evacuator
   o D. Poole suction

146. **Which type of hematoma is a result of torn bridging meningeal veins?**

o A. Subdural
o B. Epidural
o C. Intracerebral
o D. Intraventricular

147. **In addition to temperature, time and moisture, what is the fourth factor that determines the outcome of the steam sterilization process?**

o A. Concentration
o B. Aeration
o C. Weight
o D. Pressure

148. **The Bowie-Dick test is performed:**

o A. Hourly
o B. Daily
o C. Weekly
o D. Monthly

149. **The spiral, conical structure of the inner ear is the:**

o A. Cochlea
o B. Stapes
o C. Vestibule
o D. Labyrinth

150. **What is the name of the condition in which a loop of bowel herniates into the Douglas's cul-de-sac?**

o A. Cystocele
o B. Rectocele
· o C. Enterocele
o D. Omphalocele

151. **Which of these conditions is characterized by a fleshy encroachment of conjunctiva onto the cornea?**

o A. Chalazion
o B. Pterygium
o C. Strabismus
o D. Ecchymosis

152. **Which procedure would be listed in the OR schedule for a patient undergoing surgical treatment of uterine fibroids?**

o A. Pelvic exenteration
o B. Cervical cerclage
o C. Colporrhaphy
o D. Myomectomy

153. **Where is a Baker's cyst located?**

o A. Olecranon process

o B. Greater tubercle

o C. Popliteal fossa

o D. Carpal tunnel

154. **Which of the following is a method of high-level disinfection?**

o A. Peracetic acid for 30 minutes

o B. 2% glutaraldehyde for 20 minutes

o C. Steam under pressure for 10 minutes

o D. Hydrogen peroxide gas plasma for 75 minutes

155. **Another name for the tympanic membrane is the:**

o A. Ear tube

o B. Ear canal

o C. Earlobe

o D. Eardrum

156. **What is the burn degree classification that involves the epidermis and subcutaneous tissue?**

o A. First

o B. Second

o C. Third

o D. Fourth

157. **Which portion of the ear is affected by Méniére's syndrome?**

o A. Inner

o B. Middle

o C. Eustachian tube

o D. Auditory ossicles

158. **The cartilaginous nasal septum is anterior to which bone?**

o A. Hyoid

o B. Vomer

o C. Mandible

o D. Palatine

159. **The most reliable method for determining the efficiency of moist heat sterilizers is the controlled use of biological indicators containing the organism:**

o A. *Bacillus stearothermophilus*

o B. *Clostridium tetani*

o C. *Bordetella pertussis*

o D. *Corynebacterium diphtheria*

160. **Which neurosurgical pathology would a myelogram diagnose?**

   o A. Subdural hematoma
   o B. Creutzfeldt-Jakob
   o C. Spinal stenosis
   o D. Myelomeningocele

161. **Which of the following terms means a prolapsed bladder causing a bulge in the anterior vaginal wall?**

   o A. Rectocele
   o B. Cystocele
   o C. Enterocele
   o D. Herniation

162. **How many hours must the steam sterilization biological indicator incubate?**

   o A. 6
   o B. 12
   o C. 18
   o D. 24

163. **The nasal sinus located between the nose and the orbits is the:**

   o A. Frontal
   o B. Sphenoid
   o C. Ethmoid
   o D. Maxillary

164. **What is the definition of otosclerosis?**

   o A. Earache
   o B. Tinnitus
   o C. Tearing of tympanic membrane
   o D. Bony overgrowth of stapes

165. **Which of the following terms describes a fracture in which the bone penetrates the skin?**

   o A. Comminuted
   o B. Compound
   o C. Simple
   o D. Closed

166. **For which of the following procedures would a McBurney incision be indicated?**

   o A. Appendectomy
   o B. Cholecystectomy
   o C. Herniorrhaphy
   o D. Gastrectomy

167. **What degrees Celsius is the steam sterilization biological indicator incubated?**

o A. 43-48
o B. 49-54
o C. 55-60
o D. 61-66

168. **What is the medical term for removal of the uterus?**

o A. Salpingectomy
o B. Oophorectomy
o C. Myomectomy
o D. Hysterectomy

169. **Which of the following methods removes small organic particles and soil from the box locks and ratchets of instruments?**

o A. Ultrasonic washer
o B. Manual cleaning
o C. Washer-sterilizer
o D. Enzymatic soak

170. **What is the medical term for nosebleed?**

o A. Rhinitis
o B. Sinusitis
o C. Epistaxis
o D. Hemoptysis

171. **What is the proper method for preparing a Frazier suction tip for steam sterilization?**

o A. Lumen is dry
o B. Distilled water in lumen
o C. Stylet is left inside lumen
o D. Disinfectant solution in lumen

172. **Which of the following is a telescoping of the intestines in neonates requiring immediate surgical intervention?**

o A. Intussusception
o B. Pyloric stenosis
o C. Tetralogy of Fallot
o D. Omphalocele

173. **The minimum Fahrenheit temperature for sterilization to occur in a prevacuum steam sterilizer is:**

o A. 249-255
o B. 256-262
o C. 263-269
o D. 270-276

174. **What is the name of the procedure for the excision of the tunica vaginalis?**

o A. Spermatocelectomy

o B. Orchiectomy

o C. Hydrocelectomy

o D. Vasectomy

175. **What is the minimum number of minutes to sterilize unwrapped metal instruments with lumens in the gravity displacement sterilizer at 270° F?**

o A. 5

o B. 10

o C. 15

o D. 20

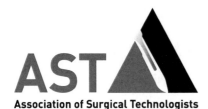
1.	A	31.	A	61.	B	91.	B	121.	B	151.	B
2.	D	32.	A	62.	A	92.	B	122.	D	152.	D
3.	B	33.	D	63.	C	93.	C	123.	C	153.	C
4.	B	34.	C	64.	A	94.	A	124.	A	154.	B
5.	D	35.	A	65.	B	95.	B	125.	B	155.	D
6.	A	36.	C	66.	B	96.	D	126.	C	156.	C
7.	C	37.	B	67.	C	97.	D	127.	B	157.	A
8.	A	38.	B	68.	A	98.	C	128.	D	158.	B
9.	A	39.	C	69.	B	99.	C	129.	C	159.	A
10.	D	40.	D	70.	C	100.	A	130.	A	160.	C
11.	A	41.	C	71.	B	101.	C	131.	C	161.	B
12.	D	42.	A	72.	A	102.	D	132.	A	162.	D
13.	B	43.	B	73.	B	103.	D	133.	C	163.	C
14.	C	44.	B	74.	D	104.	A	134.	D	164.	D
15.	B	45.	D	75.	A	105.	C	135.	B	165.	B
16.	C	46.	D	76.	B	106.	D	136.	C	166.	A
17.	A	47.	B	77.	D	107.	C	137.	B	167.	C
18.	B	48.	C	78.	C	108.	A	138.	A	168.	D
19.	C	49.	B	79.	A	109.	C	139.	C	169.	A
20.	A	50.	A	80.	B	110.	A	140.	B	170.	C
21.	D	51.	A	81.	C	111.	D	141.	C	171.	B
22.	C	52.	A	82.	A	112.	C	142.	D	172.	A
23.	A	53.	A	83.	C	113.	B	143.	A	173.	D
24.	B	54.	B	84.	B	114.	B	144.	B	174.	C
25.	B	55.	A	85.	A	115.	D	145.	C	175.	B
26.	C	56.	A	86.	B	116.	A	146.	A		
27.	A	57.	C	87.	A	117.	D	147.	D		
28.	B	58.	B	88.	B	118.	B	148.	B		
29.	A	59.	C	89.	D	119.	A	149.	A		
30.	A	60.	B	90.	A	120.	C	150.	C		

1. **A.** The teeth are located in the sockets of the alveolar processes of the mandible and maxillae.

2. **D.** Clean-contaminated procedures include those when the aerodigestive tract is entered. The bronchoscope is inserted through the mouth and into the bronchial tubes. The procedure is considered clean, not sterile.

3. **B.** Alpha-chymotrypsin is a solution used to soften the zonules holding the lens before cataract surgery to ease extraction of the lens.

4. **B.** The patient should be placed in the elevator entering head first and exit feet first when being transported to the OR on the stretcher.

5. **D.** Pfannenstiel's incision is a curved transverse incision across the lower abdomen and used frequently in gynecologic surgery.

6. **A.** Metal trays that are perforated or have a mesh bottom should be placed on the sterilizing cart flat.

7. **C.** Potassium plays four important roles: influences the electrical excitability of cells; the amount of potassium in cells affects cell volume; potassium balance is important in maintaining the acid-base balance; the amount of potassium in cells affects cell metabolism. Hyperkalemia, an abnormal level of potassium, can be life threatening, causing cardiac irregularities.

8. **A.** Curved Mayo scissors are large scissors, with thick blades used to cut tough tissue, such as fascia, tendons and muscle.

9. **A.** The argon laser beam can travel through clear fluids and tissues.

10. **D.** Informed consent must be obtained from the patient before any invasive procedure can be performed. It protects the patient because it verifies that he/she understands the condition to be treated and the intervention to be performed.

11. **A.** The cardia is the portion of the stomach that surrounds the superior opening of the stomach.

12. **D.** Low-level disinfectants kill most types of bacteria and some fungi and viruses, but do not kill spores and *M. tuberculosis.*

13. **B.** Webbing of the digits is syndactyly.

14. **C.** Surgical packs should be opened on the backtable.

15. **B.** The islets of Langerhans secrete glucagon, insulin, somatostatin and pancreatic polypeptide.

16. **C.** The removal of a tooth or teeth is an extraction procedure. The resection of the soft tissue and excision of the bone surrounding the tooth prior to the removal is called odontectomy.

17. **A.** *Escherichia coli* is a gram-negative rod that is part of the normal flora of the intestinal tract of humans and is also an opportunistic bacteria.

18. **B.** When using four towels for squaring off the incision site, the first towel will be passed when standing on the same side as the surgeon.

19. **C.** The skin is rendered surgically clean when a properly performed surgical scrub is done.

20. **A.** The pancreatic ducts join at the ampulla of Vater.

21. **D.** The patient should be identified by name, date of birth and physician on their ID bracelet prior to transporting the patient to the OR.

22. **C.** Spirilli are spiral-shaped bacteria.

23. **A.** The gallbladder stores bile until it is needed in the small intestine.

24. **B.** The circulator is not a part of the sterile team. The circulator performs his/her duties on the periphery of the sterile field.

25. **B.** Sliding doors are usually used in the OR because they eliminate air currents caused by swinging doors, but a disadvantage is they do not aid in controlling OR temperature.

26. **C.** Time relates to the length of time the surgical technologist is exposed to the ionizing radiation. Shielding means donning lead aprons and other lead shield devices for protection from the radiation. Distance means standing as far away as possible out of the path of the direct beam of ionizing radiation.

27. **A.** The duodenum starts at the pyloric sphincter of the stomach.

28. **B.** The surgical position frequently used for patients undergoing kidney surgery is the lateral position with the operative site exposed.

29. **A.** Most rickettsiae are obligate intracellular parasites. They are usually transmitted by arthropod vectors.

30. **A.** A binocular microscope is used during an examination of the vagina called a colposcopy. Colpo is a word root that means vagina.

31. **A.** Tamponade is the compression of the heart due to a collection of blood or fluid within the pericardium.

32. **A.** The anesthesia provider decides when the patient is stable and ready for transport from the OR to the PACU.

33. **D.** The suffix –centesis means surgical puncture. When combined with arthrocentesis, it means surgical puncture of a joint space with a needle to remove fluid.

34. **C.** The appendix is attached to the cecum.

35. **A.** A Gram stain determines the shape and grouping characteristics of bacteria.

36. **C.** Mydriatics are used to dilate the pupil for examination of the retina, refraction testing, or easier removal of the lens.

37. **B.** U-drape is a type of nonfenestrated split sheet. The tails are created by a U-shape in the center of the drape.

38. **B.** Never remove a patient's identification bracelet unless the patient is discharged from the facility.

39. **C.** Supine position is the optimal surgical position for a mitral valve replacement procedure.

40. **D.** The argon laser is used because the beam travels through clear tissues without heating it, making it ideal for use on retinal disorders.

41. **C.** The biological indicator (BI) contains *Bacillus stearothermophilus* which is killed when exposed to steam sterilization conditions. The BI is the only test that guarantees sterility.

42. **A.** The greater omentum is an apron-like structure that lies over the intestines.

43. **B.** Bacteria that can live without oxygen are anaerobes.

44. **B.** A fistula is an abnormal tract that is open at both ends; it most often develops after bladder, bowel and pelvic procedures.

45. **D.** An antagonist drug neutralizes or impedes the action of another drug, that is, reverses its effects.

46. **D.** Circumferential is the term that describes the type of skin prep of an entire extremity.

47. **B.** If a tumor of an ovary is found to be malignant, the surgeon will excise both ovaries, both fallopian tubes, and the uterus to ensure that all cancer cells have been removed.

48. **C.** Kyphosis is an exaggeration of the thoracic curve of the spine, resulting in a condition commonly called hunchback.

49. **B.** Hallux valgus is the medical term for a bunion, which is a bony exostosis located on the medial side of the first metatarsal head of the big toe.

50. **A.** Another name for a lower oblique incision is inguinal incision.

51. **A.** The mesentery binds the small intestine to the posterior abdominal wall.

52. **A.** Commensalism is a relationship between two organisms when one organism benefits but the second organism is not harmed.

53. **A.** Methylprednisolone acetate (Depo-Medrol®) is a steroid used topically to diminish inflammation after ophthalmic surgery.

54. **B.** A witness verifies that the patient who is illiterate marks with an "X."

55. **A.** The direction of the stretcher should be oriented feet first, side rails up when a patient is being transported to the OR on the stretcher.

56. **A.** Blood or a urine sample should be given preoperatively by a premenopausal woman to check for human chorionic gonadotropin (HCG) which is an indicator for pregnancy.

57. **C.** Gowns are considered sterile only in front from chest to level of sterile field and the sleeves 2 in. above the elbows to the cuffs.

58. **B.** A coude is a urinary catheter with a small, curved tapered tip.

59. **C.** The reverse Trendelenburg position provides good exposure of the operative site for a thyroidectomy and allows the viscera to fall away or toward the feet to provide better exposure of the gallbladder.

60. **B.** Patent ductus arteriosus is a congenital defect when the fetal blood vessel between the pulmonary artery and aorta does not close.

61. **B.** Formalin is the most common preservative solution that tissue specimens are placed in.

62. **A.** The surgeon should be immediately notified and a recount completed.

63. **C.** The parotid glands are located inferior and anterior to the ears between the skin and masseter muscle. The parotid glands are attacked by the mumps virus.

64. **A.** An event/incident report is completed by members of the surgical team that are witness to any unusual or adverse event that affected the care provided to the surgical patient.

65. **B.** The Trendelenburg position is best used for pelvic and lower abdominal procedures, such as an abdominal hysterectomy. The position allows the viscera to fall away or toward the head for better exposure of the operative site.

66. **B.** Adaptic™ is a type of nonadherent dressing that can be used as the inner layer of a three-layer dressing.

67. **C.** A fenestrated drape is a drape with an opening, such as an aperture drape commonly used to drape eyes.

68. **A.** Hernias that occur within Hesselbach's triangle and do not have a sac are a direct inguinal hernia.

69. **B.** The Kocher is a type of oblique incision used for exposing the biliary tract (right side) or spleen (left side).

70. **C.** Bakes common duct dilators are used to dilate the common bile duct during an exploration for gallstones.

71. **B.** Ligature, also called ties or stick ties when a needle is attached, are strands of suture material used to tie off a blood vessel to stop bleeding.

72. **A.** The pancreas lies posterior to the greater curvature of the stomach; its ducts join the CBD to form the ampulla of Vater.

73. **B.** The functions of the cerebellum include regulating the initiation and termination of voluntary movements of the body, regulating the muscle tone that is necessary for body movements and controling the subconscious contractions of skeletal muscles.

74. **D.** Parasitism is a relationship when an organism benefits at the expense of the host microorganisms.

75. **A.** An acute disease is one that has a rapid onset and is followed by a speedy recovery.

76. **B.** Mitochondria produce energy-rich ATP.

77. **D.** Balanced anesthesia is also known as neuroleptanesthesia.

78. **C.** The surgeon is ultimately responsible for obtaining the surgical consent.

79. **A.** The most commonly used position for neurosurgical procedures is supine since it allows exposure to the frontal, parietal and temporal lobes.

80. **B.** The serosa is the outermost layer of most portions of the gastrointestinal tract.

81. **C.** The donor site should be scrubbed with a colorless antiseptic solution, such as chlorhexidine gluconate, to allow the surgeon the ability to evaluate the vascularity of the graft postoperatively.

82. **A.** When the patient is placed in the lateral position, and a flank incision is made, a transverse drape will be used.

83. **C.** The safety strap should be placed over the thighs approximately 2 in. proximal to the knees when transporting a patient to the OR on a stretcher, or positioning on the OR table.

84. **B.** An epispadias repair is performed to correct the congenital absence of the anterior wall of the urethra and abnormal location of the urethral orifice on the dorsum of the penis.

85. **A.** The laser provides an intense and concentrated beam of light.

86. **B.** The most common cause of intracerebral hemorrhage is hypertension.

87. **A.** The larynx is a small passageway between the pharynx and the trachea.

88. **B.** Trauma is the most common cause of retinal detachment.

89. **D.** Pulmonary embolism can be caused by fat which dislodges after fracture of a long bone or pelvis, or when performing a total hip arthroplasty.

90. **A.** The Penrose drain is a passive drain made from latex that relies on gravity for wound drainage.

91. **B.** The larynx is the location of the vocal cords.

92. **B.** Vaccination is artificially acquired active immunity.

93. **C.** Cricoid pressure occludes the esophagus to prevent regurgitation.

94. **A.** A trephine is placed on the cornea to make the circular corneal cut and into the anterior chamber during a keratoplasty.

95. **B.** A minimum of four people is required. The anesthesia provider is responsible for the head and neck of the patient, one person on the side of the stretcher, one person on the side of the OR table, and a person at the end of the OR table responsible for the feet and legs.

96. **D.** Standard Precautions, as defined by the CDC in 1996, are a combination of Universal Precautions and body substance isolation rules that state all body fluids and blood should be considered infectious.

97. **D.** Separation anxiety is the major source of distress for toddler and preschool aged patients.

98. **C.** The nasopharynx is the uppermost portion of the pharynx; the middle portion of the pharynx is the oropharynx; and the lowest portion of the pharynx is the laryngopharynx.

99. **C.** Otoplasty is performed to correct a protruding auricle of the ear.

100. **A.** A patient that sustains an injury, either unintentional or intentional, caused when a healthcare provider is caring for the patient is called an iatrogenic injury.

101. **C.** The choroid is highly vascularized and provides nutrients to the posterior surface of the retina.

102. **D.** Safety refers to the patient's perception that his/her environment is safe and free from danger.

103. **D.** Abdominal aortic aneurysms occur chiefly below the renal arteries and between the renal and iliac arteries.

104. **A.** Heparinized saline is an irrigating solution used to flush the inside of an artery.

105. **C.** The bone-to-bone fixation is first accomplished followed by reanastomosis of blood vessels and nerves.

106. **D.** A full-thickness skin graft encompasses both the epidermis and dermis.

107. **C.** Skeletal muscle tissue is striated because the fibers contain alternating light and dark bands perpendicular to the long area of the fibers. It is considered voluntary, because it is controlled consciously.

108. **A.** Microtia is the medical term for absence of the external ear or auricle.

109. **C.** The tourniquet should be deflated every 1½ hours to allow blood flow into the leg and transport oxygen to prevent tissue necrosis.

110. **A.** *Clostridium perfringens* causes gas gangrene.

111. **D.** Chest rolls should span the distance bilaterally between acromioclavicular joint to iliac crest.

112. **C.** The stapes covers the opening between the middle and inner ear known as the oval window.

113. **B.** Jackknife is another name for the Kraske position.

114. **B.** Kittner dissecting sponges are small rolls of cotton tape that are tightly rolled and used by the surgeon for blunt dissection. The sponge is loaded on the tip of a clamp, such as a Kelly.

115. **D.** The Cottingham punch is used to create the correct size of the donor cornea during a keratoplasty.

116. **A.** A complete displacement of a joint or displacement of one articular surface from another is called a luxation, and a partial dislocation is called a subluxation.

117. **D.** A disorder when fatty deposits form on the walls of arteries is known as atherosclerosis.

118. **B.** Plaster rolls used in casting should be submerged in slightly lukewarm water at approximately 70-75° F.

119. **A.** The cornea is nonvascular, transparent and covers the iris.

120. **C.** Surgical masks should be changed after each case.

121. **B.** Bacillus is a rod-shaped bacteria.

122. **D.** Gas sterilizers operate at a lower temperature as compared to steam sterilizers. The gas sterilizer operates between 85-145° F.

123. **C.** If a towel clip penetrates a sterile drape, the tips of the clip must be considered contaminated, and it should not be removed until the end of the procedure.

124. **A.** Res ipsa loquitur means "the thing speaks for itself." It refers to the harm to the patient resulting from a given act when the caregiver had sole control.

125. **B.** The glottis is the space between the vocal cords.

126. **C.** *Clostridium tetani* could possibly be found in a penetrating wound, caused by a rusty nail.

127. **B.** The Love nerve root retractor is used during spinal procedures, such as a laminectomy to gently retract the nerve roots.

128. **D.** Another name for the electrosurgical unit's patient return electrode is grounding pad.

129. **C.** 16 Fr is the size of a Foley catheter commonly used on adults.

130. **A.** A tumor arising from the covering of the brain is a meningioma.

131. **C.** The sclera gives shape to the eyeball and makes it more rigid.

132. **A.** Flagella are fine, thread-like appendages that provide bacteria with motion.

133. **C.** The Trendelenburg position allows the viscera to fall away or toward the head providing better exposure of the operative site when performing a lower abdominal or pelvic procedure.

134. **D.** Glutaraldehyde is a liquid disinfecting and sterilizing agent. To sterilize an item, it must be submersed for 10 hours.

135. **B.** Blood pressure is measured in two numbers, systolic over diastolic. The relaxation phase of the heart beat is called the diastolic blood pressure.

136. **C.** Cerumen is another term for earwax.

137. **B.** The auditory ossicles of the middle ear are the malleus, incus and stapes.

138. **A.** Exsanguination is the term for the process of removing blood from an extremity.

139. **C.** The nasolacrimal duct carries the lacrimal fluid and tears into the nasal cavity. The duct can become obstructed in pediatric patients who experience chronic URIs.

140. **B.** The surgical technologist is responsible for setting up the sterile field.

141. **C.** Cell saver transfusion cannot be used in the presence of cancer cells, gross contamination or infections.

142. **D.** Intraluminal staplers are used to anastomose tubular organs in the gastrointestinal tract. They are often used during resection and reanastomosis of the colon or rectum.

143. **A.** Satinsky, Herrick and Mayo clamps are commonly used during procedures on the kidney. Specifically, they are clamped onto the kidney pedicle.

144. **B.** The nasal cavity is divided into right and left sides by the nasal septum.

145. **C.** The Ellik evacuator is filled with irrigation solution by the first scrub surgical technologist. It is used by the surgeon for the irrigation/ evacuation of the bladder to remove prostatic tissue during a TURP.

146. **A.** A subdural hematoma is a large, encapsulated collection of blood over one or both cerebral hemispheres that causes intracranial pressure.

147. **D.** The four factors of steam sterilization are pressure, temperature, moisture and time. Pressure is used to increase the temperature of the steam to the level where it will kill microbes including spores.

148. **B.** The Bowie-Dick test is only used for pre-vacuum sterilizers to check for air entrapment and is conducted daily.

149. **A.** The cochlea is a bony spiral canal in the ear.

150. **C.** An enterocele is a herniation of Douglas's cul-de-sac that usually contains loops of the bowel.

151. **B.** Pterygium is a fleshy encroachment of conjunctiva on the cornea.

152. **D.** A myomectomy is the procedure performed for the removal of fibromyomas or fibroid tumors from the uterine wall.

153. **C.** Baker's cysts affect the popliteal fossa.

154. **B.** 2% glutaraldehyde is a type of high-level disinfectant solution. The device must be completely submersed for 20 minutes at room temperature in order to be disinfected.

155. **D.** The eardrum is also referred to as the tympanic membrane.

156. **C.** The skin, along with its epithelial structures and subcutaneous tissue, is destroyed in a third-degree burn.

157. **A.** Méniére's syndrome involves an increased amount of endolymph that enlarges the membranous labyrinth, located in the inner ear.

158. **B.** The vomer forms the inferior and posterior parts of the nasal septum.

159. **A.** *B. stearothermophilus*, in spore form, is highly resistant to destruction by steam sterilization, but does not cause disease in humans.

160. **C.** A myelogram is a diagnostic procedure when radiopaque dye is injected into the spinal subarachnoid space through a lumbar puncture. The myelogram would diagnose spinal stenosis.

161. **B.** A cystocele is a herniation of the bladder that causes a downward bulge in the anterior vaginal wall, usually as a result of surgical trauma, age, or weakness of the supporting muscles of the bladder due to childbirth.

162. **D.** The steam sterilization biological indicator must be incubated for 24 hours before the reading is recorded.

163. **C.** The ethmoid sinus is located between the nose and orbits.

164. **D.** Otosclerosis is the formation and hardening of spongy bone in the ear.

165. **B.** A compound or open fracture is one when the bone has penetrated the skin layer and protrudes through the opening.

166. **A.** The McBurney incision is primarily used for removal of the appendix.

167. **C.** The steam biological indicator must be incubated at a temperature of 55-60° C.

168. **D.** Hysterectomy is the medical term that means removal of the uterus. Hyster is the root word that means "uterus;" -ectomy is a suffix meaning "removal or excision of."

169. **A.** The ultrasonic cleaner uses the process of cavitation to remove small organic particles and soil from the areas of instrumentation that can't be accomplished through manual or mechanical cleaning.

170. **C.** Epistaxis is the medical term for nosebleed.

171. **B.** Air trapped in the lumen will prevent steam from contacting the inner surface of the lumen. A residual amount of distilled water should be left inside the lumen which will boil and turn to steam to displace the air.

172. **A.** Intussusception is the most common emergency surgery for neonates when the portion of the bowel slides into another segment and causes obstruction. The motion is like a telescope.

173. **D.** The minimum Farenheit temperature for items to be rendered sterile is 270–276° F.

174. **C.** Excision of the tunica vaginalis of the testis is called a hydrocelectomy.

175. **B.** When immediate-use sterilization (formerly called "flash sterilization") is used to sterilize items with lumens in the gravity sterilizer, the items must be exposed to 270° F for 10 minutes.

AST

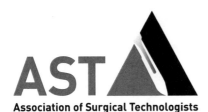

ASSOCIATION OF SURGICAL TECHNOLOGISTS

PRACTICE EXAM #2 FOR CERTIFICATION EXAMINATION

Directions: *Be sure to read each question carefully and select the best answer. You have four hours to complete the test. After finishing the test, review the answers and score your exam.*

In order to pass the CST examination, you must answer 118 questions correctly. If you achieved that score—congratulations! If not, take the time to identify what topics you struggled with and review the appropriate material.

---

1. **Which of the following is a type of tissue forceps?**

   o A. Brown-Adson

   o B. Pean

   o C. Allis

   o D. Schnidt

2. **Which endoscope is used to visualize the heart and major vessels?**

   o A. Ventriculoscope

   o B. Bronchoscope

   o C. Mediastinoscope

   o D. Angioscope

3. **The goal of the surgical scrub is to lower the population of which flora to an irreducible minimum?**

   o A. Parasitic

   o B. Resident

   o C. Transient

   o D. Enteric

4. **Which needle is used during the bladder suspension procedure for treating stress incontinence in women?**

   o A. Stamey

   o B. Chiba

   o C. Dorsey

   o D. Tru-Cut

5. **Which procedure can be performed without making an incision to treat varicose veins?**

   o A. Sclerotherapy

   o B. Varicocelectomy

   o C. Vein ligation

   o D. Vein stripping

6. When repairing a direct hernia, the surgeon works within the anatomical triangle formed by the inguinal ligament, inferior epigastric vessels and the lateral border of the rectus abdominis called:

   o A. Femoral

   o B. Anterior

   o C. Hesselbach's

   o D. Calot's

7. Which of the following is the correct postoperative sequence of actions completed by the surgical technologist?
   1. Assist with postoperative patient care
   2. Remove drapes
   3. Remove gown and gloves
   4. Break down sterile setup

   o A. 2, 1, 4, 3

   o B. 2, 3, 1, 4

   o C. 3, 2, 4, 1

   o D. 4, 2, 1, 3

8. What should be completed before the sterile items are opened for the first procedure of the day?

   o A. Lower temperature in the OR

   o B. Wipe down furniture and surfaces

   o C. Test sterilizer in substerile room

   o D. Test anesthesia machine

9. Cardiac muscles are controlled by which division of the nervous system?

   o A. Sympathetic

   o B. Somatic

   o C. Autonomic

   o D. Central

10. Oophor/o is the root word for which anatomical structure?

    o A. Ovary

    o B. Uterus

    o C. Cervical os

    o D. Fallopian tube

11. In which of the following would absorbable suture be contraindicated?

    o A. Peritoneum

    o B. Muscle

    o C. Intestinal anastomosis

    o D. Vascular anastomosis

12. **During a cesarean section, which organ is freed from the uterus to prevent injury?**

o A. Pelvic ligaments

o B. Ureters

o C. Fallopian tubes

o D. Bladder

13. **Which of the following refers to the absence of pathogens?**

o A. Pathological

o B. Aseptic

o C. Septic

o D. Nosocomial

14. **Which surgical procedure would use the instrument shown below ?**

o A. D&C

o B. Colporrhaphy

o C. LAVH

o D. Myomectomy

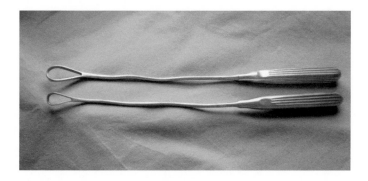

15. **What must be done prior to positioning a patient undergoing a posterior lumbar laminectomy?**

o A. Attachment of arm boards

o B. Padding of knees

o C. Endotracheal intubation

o D. Skin prep

16. **What is the name of the instrument shown below?**

    o A. Carmalt
    o B. Ochsner
    o C. Adair
    o D. Pennington

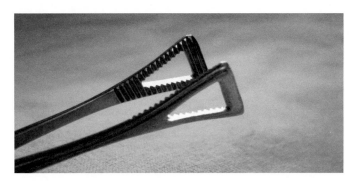

17. **Which of the following damages the mastoid air cells and ossicles of the ear?**

    o A. Meniere's disease
    o B. Acoustic neuroma
    o C. Cholesteatoma
    o D. Otosclerosis

18. **When placing a swaged needle onto a needle holder, the needle should be clamped:**

    o A. One-third distance from swaged end of needle
    o B. One-fourth distance from the needle point
    o C. At the junction of suture and needle
    o D. Half-way distance from the needle point

19. **Which endoscope is used for the removal of foreign bodies from the airway of a pediatric patient?**

    o A. Flexible esophagoscope
    o B. Flexible bronchoscope
    o C. Rigid esophagoscope
    o D. Rigid bronchoscope

20. **Which of the following elements primarily make up the body's mass?**

    o A. Oxygen, carbon, magnesium, sodium
    o B. Oxygen, potassium, hydrogen, sulfur
    o C. Oxygen, carbon, hydrogen, nitrogen
    o D. Oxygen, carbon, phosphorus, magnesium

21.   **Which instrument is used to contract the ribs for suturing purposes?**

o A.   Bailey

o B.   Semb

o C.   Matson

o D.   Doyen

22.   **The largest muscle of the upper calf is the:**

o A.   Tibialis

o B.   Peroneus

o C.   Gastrocnemius

o D.   Quadriceps

23.   **What is the length of time when thrombin loses its potency?**

o A.   30 minutes

o B.   60 minutes

o C.   2 hours

o D.   3 hours

24.   **The function of the small intestine is:**

o A.   Synthesis of vitamins

o B.   Absorption of nutrients

o C.   Production of bacteria

o D.   Excretion of bile

25.   **The teeth are composed primarily of:**

o A.   Dentin

o B.   Cementum

o C.   Enamel

o D.   Pulp

26.   **The basis for the design of electrical equipment in the OR is:**

o A.   Alternating current

o B.   Isolated circuit

o C.   Electron theory

o D.   Ohm's Law

27.   **Which of the following procedures is performed to decrease gastric secretions?**

o A.   Pyloroplasty

o B.   Vagotomy

o C.   Billroth I

o D.   Gastrostomy

28. **A patient who underwent an appendectomy enters the emergency department with severe abdominal pain, constipation and vomiting. Which of the following is occurring?**

   o   A.   Cholecystitis
   o   B.   Obstructed bowel
   o   C.   Diverticulitis
   o   D.   Strangulated hernia

29. **Which organ shares the same blood supply with the pancreas and must be removed during a Whipple procedure?**

   o   A.   Kidney
   o   B.   Duodenum
   o   C.   Bladder
   o   D.   Spleen

30. **During a cleft palate procedure, which equipment should the surgical technologist be prepared to set up quickly?**

   o   A.   Drill
   o   B.   Microscope
   o   C.   Nerve stimulator
   o   D.   Saw

31. **The muscle that flexes and supinates the forearm and covers the anterior portion of the upper arm is the:**

   o   A.   Flexor radialis
   o   B.   Biceps brachii
   o   C.   Brachioradialis
   o   D.   Teres major

32. **A surgeon tells a patient she has terminal cancer but requires prophylactic surgery to prevent a bowel obstruction and the patient replies, "This can't be happening to me." Which stage of grief is the patient displaying?**

   o   A.   Denial
   o   B.   Depression
   o   C.   Bargaining
   o   D.   Anger

33. **What is the purpose of inserting a ureteral stent catheter?**

   o   A.   Monitor urine output
   o   B.   Bypass calculi obstruction
   o   C.   Excise calculi
   o   D.   Prevent postoperative hemorrhage

34. **Which of the following is used to create the trough on the anterior glenoid rim during a Bankart procedure?**

o A. Periosteal elevator

o B. Bone cutting forceps

o C. Shaver with abrader tip

o D. Reciprocating saw

35. **Which of the following secretes hydrochloric acid?**

o A. Parietal cells

o B. Salivary glands

o C. Pancreas

o D. Duodenum

36. **Which of the following preoperative diagnostic tests would be administered to a patient with a brain injury?**

o A. EEG

o B. EMG

o C. SAO2

o D. TEE

37. **Which of the following is a type of fenestrated drape?**

o A. Incise

o B. Three-quarter

o C. Extremity

o D. Split

38. **The walls of the vagina are lined with:**

o A. Fascia

o B. Mucosa

o C. Serosa

o D. Peritoneum

39. **Which type of scalpel uses ultrasonic energy to cut and coagulate tissue?**

o A. Fulguration

o B. Hemostatic

o C. Harmonic

o D. Plasma

40. **A Fogarty catheter is used during a/an:**

o A. Gastrectomy

o B. Thoracotomy

o C. Embolectomy

o D. Craniotomy

41. **Which of the following positioning devices is needed when placing the patient in the supine position?**

   o A. Kidney rest

   o B. Elbow pads

   o C. Mayfield headrest

   o D. Beanbag

42. **During a trabeculectomy, which two layers are incised at the beginning of the procedure?**

   o A. Cornea; iris

   o B. Pupil; lens

   o C. Conjunctiva; Tenon's capsule

   o D. Sclera; retina

43. **What instrument set should the surgical technologist have available in the OR when preparing for an inguinal herniorraphy?**

   o A. Rectal

   o B. Bowel

   o C. Vascular

   o D. Biliary

44. **Which of the following is used to obtain specimens during a bronchoscopy?**

   o A. Test tube

   o B. Suction container

   o C. Lukens tube

   o D. 4x4 Raytec sponges

45. **Which suture material would be used in the presence of infection?**

   o A. Polyglycolic acid

   o B. Silk

   o C. Chromic gut

   o D. Steel

46. **Which surgical procedure uses the instrument shown below?**

    o   A.   Vulvectomy
    o   B.   Meniscectomy
    o   C.   Laminectomy
    o   D.   Blepharoplasty

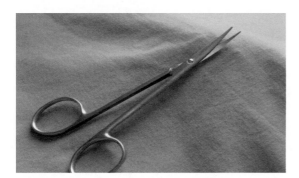

47. **Which surgical specialty most often uses the instrument shown below?**

    o   A.   Gynecologic
    o   B.   Genitourinary
    o   C.   Maxillofacial
    o   D.   Orthopedic

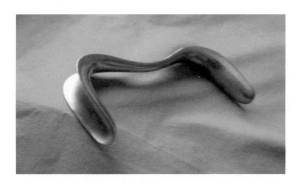

48. **Which of the following hernias can result in necrosis of the viscera?**

    o   A.   Irreducible
    o   B.   Strangulated
    o   C.   Femoral
    o   D.   Sliding

49. **When the surgeon makes a McBurney's incision, which muscle is encountered first and divided in the direction of its fibers?**

    o   A.   Transverse abdominis
    o   B.   Rectus abdominis
    o   C.   Internal oblique
    o   D.   External oblique

50. **Which of the following maintains the position of the uterus?**

   o A. Suspensory ligament
   o B. Levator muscle
   o C. Broad ligament
   o D. Pubic symphysis

51. **Transverse colectomy is incised through which incision?**

   o A. Upper midline
   o B. Oblique
   o C. Paramedian
   o D. Thoracoabdominal

52. **Which kind of uterine tissue can grow in abnormal locations including the ovaries, pelvic peritoneum and small intestine?**

   o A. Perimetrial
   o B. Cervical
   o C. Endometrial
   o D. Myometrial

53. **Which preoperative diagnostic exam is quickly completed to confirm ectopic pregnancy?**

   o A. Colposcopy
   o B. Fluoroscopy
   o C. Ultrasound
   o D. MRI

54. **How would you position a patient with an intertrochanteric fracture?**

   o A. Lateral
   o B. Prone
   o C. Supine
   o D. Trendelenburg

55. **What position allows optimal exposure of the retroperitoneal area of the flank?**

   o A. Prone
   o B. Trendelenburg
   o C. Supine
   o D. Lateral

56. **Which of the following is the correct sequence of instruments for placing a screw into bone?**
    1. Depth gauge
    2. Drill
    3. Screw driver
    4. Tap

    o A. 2, 1, 4, 3
    o B. 1, 2, 4, 3
    o C. 4, 1, 2, 3
    o D. 2, 4, 1, 3

57. **The removal of fibrous thickening of the visceral pleura is:**

    o A. Pericardiectomy
    o B. Poudrage
    o C. Decortication
    o D. Segmentectomy

58. **The only depolarizing muscle relaxant in clinical use is:**

    o A. Cisatracurium (Nimbex®)
    o B. Vecuronium (Norcuron®)
    o C. Rocuronium (Zemuron®)
    o D. Succinylcholine (Anectine®)

59. **What type of hernia involves a direct and indirect inguinal hernia?**

    o A. Reducible
    o B. Umbilical
    o C. Epigastric
    o D. Pantaloon

60. **How are the legs of the patient positioned for lateral position?**

    o A. Lower leg straight; upper leg flexed
    o B. Lower leg flexed; upper leg straight
    o C. Both legs straight
    o D. Both legs flexed

61. **The neuroglia of the nervous system:**

    o A. Produce CSF
    o B. Support and bind
    o C. Conduct impulses
    o D. Initiate reflexes

62. **The method of inhalation anesthesia that allows complete rebreathing of expired gases is:**

    o A. Mask inhalation
    o B. Closed
    o C. Semi-closed
    o D. Open

63. **Which member of the surgical team is responsible for protecting an unsplinted fracture during positioning?**

    o   A.   Circulator
    o   B.   Surgical technologist preceptor
    o   C.   Surgeon
    o   D.   Anesthesia provider

64. **What personal protective equipment should the surgical technologist don prior to the start of an extracorporeal shock-wave lithotripsy procedure?**

    o   A.   Fluid proof apron
    o   B.   Eye protection
    o   C.   Non-sterile gloves
    o   D.   Lead apron

65. **Another name for tonsil suction is:**

    o   A.   Poole
    o   B.   Baron
    o   C.   Frazier
    o   D.   Yankauer

66. **Which muscles relax when a small pad is placed under a patient's head in the supine position?**

    o   A.   Cremaster
    o   B.   Deltoid
    o   C.   Strap
    o   D.   Pyramidal

67. **When a medication or local anesthetic is passed to the surgeon, the surgical technologist should:**

    o   A.   Show the surgeon the medicine bottle
    o   B.   State how much medication the circulator dispensed
    o   C.   Hand the syringe to the surgeon with the cap on the needle for safety
    o   D.   State the name and dosage of the medication

68. **A type of bone-holding forceps is:**

    o   A.   Dingman
    o   B.   Langenbeck
    o   C.   Smillie
    o   D.   Slocum

69. **Which surgical procedure would use the instrument shown below?**

o A. Endarterectomy

o B. Thoracoscopy

o C. Lobectomy

o D. Coronary artery bypass

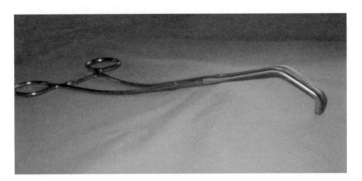

70. **According to OSHA standards, protective eyewear of some form must be worn:**

o A. Only for known HIV and HBV cases

o B. Only for cases when excessive bleeding is expected

o C. On orthopedic cases only

o D. On all cases

71. **Which pathological condition of the small intestine could be misdiagnosed as acute appendicitis?**

o A. Gastritis

o B. Carcinoma

o C. Crohn's disease

o D. Meckel's diverticulum

72. **Which piece of equipment is required for administration of a Bier block?**

o A. Pulse oximeter

o B. Pain control anesthesia pump

o C. Double-cuffed tourniquet

o D. Electrosurgical unit

73. **Which subcategory of drug preparation is a combination of two liquids that cannot mix?**

o A. Solution

o B. Emulsion

o C. Suspension

o D. Semisolid

74. **What is the average normal respiration rate for children?**

   o A. 10 to 17
   o B. 18 to 30
   o C. 30 to 40
   o D. 40 to 50

75. **The introduction of radiopaque contrast medium into an artery or vein is called a/an:**

   o A. Ultrasonography
   o B. Angiography
   o C. Cholangiography
   o D. Echocardiography

76. **What anatomical structure must be approximated after a colectomy to prevent herniation of abdominal contents?**

   o A. Omentum
   o B. Pylorus
   o C. Mesentery
   o D. Jejunum

77. **To prevent density, instrument sets should not exceed:**

   o A. 15 lbs
   o B. 20 lbs
   o C. 25 lbs
   o D. 10 lbs

78. **When surgically treating hydrocephalus, where is the shunt placed?**

   o A. Third ventricle
   o B. Lateral ventricle
   o C. Aqueduct of Sylvius
   o D. Foramen of Monro

79. **Which of the following is a type of uterine fibroid?**

   o A. Endometrium
   o B. Cystocele
   o C. Leiomyoma
   o D. Rectocele

80. **The ureters enter the bladder medially:**

   o A. At the distal aspect
   o B. At the superior aspect
   o C. From the posterior aspect
   o D. From the anterior aspect

81. **The pathogen that most often causes postoperative surgical site infections is:**

   o A. *Pseudomonas aeruginosa*
   o B. *Escherichia coli*
   o C. *Candida albicans*
   o D. *Staphylococcus aureus*

82. **Which organ is the most frequently injured during a motor vehicle accident?**

   o A. Spleen
   o B. Liver
   o C. Kidney
   o D. Heart

83. **Where would the surgical technologist find pertinent information for "pulling" a case?**

   o A. Laboratory reports
   o B. Surgical consent
   o C. Preference card
   o D. Hospital medical records

84. **Suture material that becomes encapsulated by fibrous tissue during the healing stage is:**

   o A. Multifilament
   o B. Fascia lata
   o C. Ligatures
   o D. Non-absorbable

85. **If a mentoplasty is being performed, the surgical technologist should confirm a prosthesis is available for the:**

   o A. Ear
   o B. Chin
   o C. Forehead
   o D. Nose

86. **Which of the following means cell "eating?"**

   o A. Phagocytosis
   o B. Filtration
   o C. Pinocytosis
   o D. Osmosis

87. **Which nerve could be damaged when the patient is placed in Fowler's position?**

   o A. Ulnar
   o B. Femoral
   o C. Brachial
   o D. Sciatic

88. **What is the correct order for donning OR attire?**
    1. Scrub suit
    2. Shoe covers
    3. Hair cover
    4. Mask

    o A. 4, 3, 1, 2
    o B. 2, 3, 1, 4
    o C. 1, 3, 4, 2
    o D. 3, 1, 4, 2

89. **The cranial nerve responsible for hearing and balance is the:**

    o A. V
    o B. VIII
    o C. XI
    o D. XII

90. **Which of the following is not a hemostatic agent used in orthopedic surgery?**

    o A. Bone wax
    o B. Gelfoam
    o C. Xeroform
    o D. Thrombin

91. **Which of the following is responsible for disseminated intravascular coagulation?**

    o A. Endotoxin
    o B. Exotoxin
    o C. Neurotoxin
    o D. Enterotoxin

92. **The copper wire in the electrosurgical unit that allows the flow of free electrons is called the:**

    o A. Resistor
    o B. Ground wire
    o C. Conductor
    o D. Insulator

93. **At the end of a procedure, the surgeon asks for the local anesthetic to inject intra-articular. Where is the surgeon injecting the local drug?**

    o A. Subcutaneous
    o B. Dermal
    o C. Within joint
    o D. Intravenous

94. **Which preoperative diagnostic test is useful in diabetic patients with small vessel arterial disease?**

o A. Plethysmography

o B. Echocardiography

o C. Capnography

o D. Isotope scanning

95. **Which of the following is the most effective method for sterilizing items that can be damaged by steam sterilization?**

o A. Plasma sterilization

o B. Ethylene oxide

o C. Glutaraldehyde

o D. Peracetic acid

96. **The mandible articulates with which bone?**

o A. Ethmoid

o B. Maxillae

o C. Temporal

o D. Zygomatic

97. **What could result from crossing the patient's arms across his/her chest in the supine position?**

o A. Interference with circulation

o B. Interference with respiration

o C. Postoperative discomfort

o D. Pressure on the median nerve

98. **Which of the following is incorrect when preparing a paper-plastic peel pack?**

o A. Ring handles of clamps are placed at end

o B. Instruments are held together with autoclave tape within the peel pack

o C. Open end of peel pack is sealed with autoclave tape

o D. Inner peel pack of a double peel pack is not sealed

99. **Which of the following degrees in Celsius equals 98.6 degrees Fahrenheit?**

o A. 34

o B. 37

o C. 30

o D. 40

100. **When the surgical technologist is preparing surgical instruments for transport to the decontamination room, which statement is incorrect?**

o A. Instruments with multiple parts should be assembled

o B. Instruments with ratchets should be unratcheted

o C. String instruments with ring handles

o D. Heavy instruments should be placed on tray bottom

101. **If a short bone is being removed from the wrist due to arthritis, what is being removed?**

    o   A.   Carpal
    o   B.   Rib
    o   C.   Tibia
    o   D.   Patella

102. **Which of the following heals by contraction, granulation and connective tissue?**

    o   A.   Primary union
    o   B.   Delayed closure
    o   C.   Maturation
    o   D.   Proliferation

103. **Before transporting instruments to the decontamination room, what should the surgical technologist complete?**

    o   A.   Confirm instruments are dry
    o   B.   Presoak instruments in detergent solution
    o   C.   Wipe off instruments with towel
    o   D.   Rinse instruments with saline

104. **Which solution is best for presoaking instruments in the OR at the end of a procedure?**

    o   A.   Iodine-based
    o   B.   Sterile water
    o   C.   Enzyme
    o   D.   Saline

105. **A mesh that is contraindicated in the presence of infection is:**

    o   A.   Vicryl™
    o   B.   Stainless steel
    o   C.   Prolene™
    o   D.   PTFE

106. **Which of the following provides additional protection to prevent contamination of a sterile package?**

    o   A.   Dust cover
    o   B.   Green towel
    o   C.   Non-sterile 3/4 sheet
    o   D.   Muslin wrap

107. **The stripes on steam chemical indicators change to what color upon exposure to sterilization parameters?**

    o   A.   Black
    o   B.   Red
    o   C.   Yellow
    o   D.   No change

108. **For which fracture is the instrument shown below best used?**

o A. Scapula
o B. Radius
o C. Calcaneus
o D. Femoral

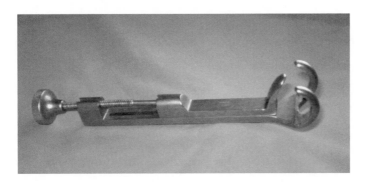

109. **During a kidney transplant, the renal vein of the donor kidney is anastomosed to the:**

o A. Superior mesenteric vein
o B. External iliac vein
o C. Inferior vena cava
o D. Hepatic portal vein

110. **Which procedure corrects testicular torsion?**

o A. Meatoplasty
o B. Orchiopexy
o C. Cystectomy
o D. Hydrocelectomy

111. **Which instrument is used to incise the tympanic membrane?**

o A. Alligator forceps
o B. Iris scissors
o C. Farrel applicator
o D. Myringotomy knife

112. **An example of a nonadherent inner layer dressing is:**

o A. Xeroform™
o B. ABD
o C. Stockinette
o D. Coban™

113. **To prevent a cerebral aneurysm from rupturing, the surgeon will:**

o A. Apply a specially designed clip at base of aneurysm
o B. Apply hemoclips on the feeder veins
o C. Incise the wall of the aneurysm
o D. Insert a Gore-Tex® graft

114. **The ophthalmologist tells the surgical technologist to place 2 drops atropine sulfate OU. What does this mean?**

    o A. Both eyes dilated
    o B. Left eye is to be dilated
    o C. Both eyes irrigated postoperatively
    o D. Right eye is to be dilated

115. **If a patient requests to see a member of the clergy upon arrival to preoperative holding:**

    o A. Call for a clergy person before the anesthesia is administered
    o B. Reassure the patient that he/she will be just fine
    o C. Have a clergy person wait for the patient in the recovery room
    o D. Chart the request and leave it to the floor personnel

116. **If cultures cannot be immediately transported from the surgery department to pathology, they should be:**

    o A. Placed in an incubator
    o B. Placed in a refrigerator
    o C. Kept at room temperature
    o D. Submerged in media

117. **In terms of transmitting an infection, what is a fomite?**

    o A. Microorganism
    o B. Inanimate object
    o C. Parasite
    o D. Active carrier

118. **When positioning the patient for a cesarean section, where is the bolster placed and why?**

    o A. Right side; relieve pressure on vena cava
    o B. Left side; relieve pressure on abdominal aorta
    o C. Pelvis; relieve pressure on sciatic nerve
    o D. Lumbar region; relieve pressure on lumbar nerves

119. **The conducting fibers that extend from the AV node to the interventricular septum form the:**

    o A. SA node
    o B. Bundle of His
    o C. Vagus bundle
    o D. Left bundle branch

120. **Items that are impenetrable to X-rays are described as:**

    o A. Radiotransparent
    o B. Radioactive
    o C. Radioresistant
    o D. Radiopaque

121. **During surgical rotation, the skills of a surgical technology student may be evaluated by the:**

o A. Certified nurse assistant
o B. Surgical technologist preceptor
o C. Director of nursing
o D. Anesthesia provider

122. **During a TRAM procedure, which is used to identify and preserve the superior epigastric arteries?**

o A. C-arm
o B. Doppler
o C. Echocardiography
o D. Angiography

123. **Which of the following should be accomplished when preparing an Esmarch bandage for sterilization?**

o A. Folded in layers
o B. Layer of Webril™ rolled with bandage
o C. Tightly rolled
o D. Unfolded mound wrapped in green towel

124. **Which of the following is the correct order of the layers of the colon?**
1. Serosa
2. Submucosa
3. Muscularis
4. Mucosa

o A. 3, 1, 4, 2
o B. 1, 2, 4, 3
o C. 4, 2, 3, 1
o D. 2, 4, 1, 3

125. **Air or fluid accumulation due to poorly approximated wound edges could result in:**

o A. Evisceration
o B. Proud flesh
o C. Ischemia
o D. Dead space

126. **What is the first step of opening a small, sterile wrapped package when establishing the sterile field?**

o A. Open all flaps simultaneously
o B. Open first flap towards self
o C. Open first flap away from self
o D. Open side flaps

127. **Which surgical approach is often used for a craniotomy for aneurysm repair?**

- o A. Temporolateral
- o B. Transphenoidal
- o C. Posterior fossa
- o D. Frontotemporal

128. **Which of the following forceps would be used during a splenectomy?**

- o A. Doyen
- o B. Randall
- o C. Right angle
- o D. Kocher

129. **A blood pH of 7.5 indicates:**

- o A. Ketosis
- o B. Normal
- o C. Alkalosis
- o D. Acidosis

130. **Which knife blade should be placed on the knife handle when preparing the Mayo stand for a knee arthroscopy?**

- o A. #10
- o B. #20
- o C. #12
- o D. #11

131. **What is the function of phagocytic white blood cells?**

- o A. Promote ribosome function
- o B. Absorb and digest food particles
- o C. Engulf and destroy bacteria
- o D. Encourage cell rejuvenation

132. **A surgical technologist is talking with a patient in the PACU with arms folded and at a distance. This could be interpreted by the patient as:**

- o A. Active listening by CST
- o B. Negative
- o C. CST is open-minded
- o D. Positive

133. **Which of the following describes the action of histamine (H_2 blockers)?**

- o A. Increase blood flow to the heart
- o B. Produce skeletal muscle relaxation
- o C. Reverse narcotic effects
- o D. Decrease gastric volume in the stomach

134. **What decision should the OR team make when treating a minor who requires a blood transfusion, but the family religion is Jehovah's Witness?**

o   A.   Do not give transfusion

o   B.   Two physicians sign consent for transfusion

o   C.   Give transfusion

o   D.   Obtain court order to provide transfusion

135. **What does 'x' equal in the proportion 3:5 = 9:x?**

o   A.   10

o   B.   15

o   C.   20

o   D.   25

136. **Which surgical procedure uses the instrument shown below?**

o   A.   Thoracotomy

o   B.   Abdominal hysterectomy

o   C.   Total hip arthroplasty

o   D.   Gastrectomy

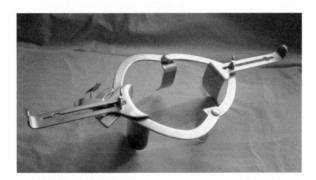

137. **During a suprapubic prostatectomy, which needle holder may be used when reconstructing the bladder outlet?**

o   A.   Heaney

o   B.   Crile-Wood

o   C.   Ryder

o   D.   Mayo-Hegar

138. **When performing a total knee arthroplasty, the surgeon removes the osteophytes from the rim of the femur and tibia with a:**

o   A.   Lambotte

o   B.   Saw

o   C.   Rasp

o   D.   Kerrison

139. **Which suture technique provides an excellent cosmetic closure?**

   o   A.   Retention
   o   B.   Reverse mattress
   o   C.   Purse-string
   o   D.   Subcuticular

140. **During a radical neck dissection with mandibulectomy, which bone is harvested for the graft?**

   o   A.   Tibia
   o   B.   Fibula
   o   C.   Ulna
   o   D.   Pelvic crest

141. **To prevent charring of bone when it is being cut or drilled, the surgical technologist should use:**

   o   A.   Irrigation/aspiration unit
   o   B.   Syringe
   o   C.   Pulse lavage
   o   D.   Suction irrigator

142. **Pain, heat, redness and swelling indicate which of the following conditions?**

   o   A.   Inflammation
   o   B.   Necrosis
   o   C.   Sepsis
   o   D.   Infection

143. **Which clamp is most often used to grasp the appendix?**

   o   A.   Dennis
   o   B.   Pean
   o   C.   Allis
   o   D.   Babcock

144. **The inner lining of the uterus is the:**

   o   A.   Perineum
   o   B.   Endometrium
   o   C.   Myometrium
   o   D.   Peritoneum

145. **Which type of dressing washes or wears off after several days?**

   o   A.   Stent
   o   B.   Steri-Strips™
   o   C.   Collodion
   o   D.   Bioclusive®

146. **A patient requires a stat cesarean section. Which of the following might be omitted?**

   o A. Protective eyewear
   o B. Counts
   o C. Donning sterile gown
   o D. Draping

147. **Which of the following is the first action to be taken following a needle stick?**

   o A. Report incident
   o B. Remove needle from the sterile field
   o C. Remove both gloves immediately
   o D. Schedule baseline testing

148. **Which of the following drapes is used for a thyroidectomy?**

   o A. Aperture
   o B. Transverse
   o C. U-drape
   o D. Incise

149. **Testosterone is secreted by the:**

   o A. Epididymis
   o B. Leydig cells
   o C. Somatic cells
   o D. Seminal vesicles

150. **When a surgeon is using a Kocher subcostal incision, which muscle is divided by electrosurgery?**

   o A. Linea alba
   o B. Rectus abdominis
   o C. Teres major
   o D. Psoas major

151. **What are the boundaries of the skin prep for a total hip arthroplasty?**

   o A. Hip region
   o B. Level of umbilicus to mid-thigh
   o C. Level of iliac crest to foot
   o D. Level of umbilicus to foot

152. **Which of the following are abdominal skin prep perimeters for an exploratory laparotomy?**

   o A. Nipple line to umbilicus
   o B. Shoulders to umbilicus
   o C. Shoulders to midthigh
   o D. Nipple line to midthigh

153. Which of the following is the main reason for wearing the OR attire?

    o A. Contain body moisture

    o B. Limit spread of microbes

    o C. Prevent strike-through

    o D. Provide comfortable attire

154. Which of the following substances are absorbed in the stomach?

    o A. Fiber

    o B. Protein

    o C. Starch

    o D. Alcohol

155. A laparotomy drape is placed on the left side inguinal area of the patient, but should have been placed on the right side. What should be done to correct the error?

    o A. Cover drape with a new drape

    o B. Remove drape and place new drape on right side

    o C. Move drape to right side

    o D. Cut opening in drape on right side

156. Which stapling device would be used during an esophagectomy to divide the esophagus?

    o A. Surgiclip™

    o B. EEA

    o C. GIA

    o D. TA

157. Movement disorder diseases caused by radiation therapy are characterized by destruction of the:

    o A. Myelin sheath

    o B. Neurofibrils

    o C. Nissl bodies

    o D. Gray matter

158. During which procedure would a Gigli saw possibly be used?

    o A. Craniotomy

    o B. Laminectomy

    o C. Acromioplasty

    o D. Bunionectomy

159. A surgeon indicates that she may place a shunt during a carotid endarterectomy. What should the surgical technologist have available in the OR?

    o A. Ventricular

    o B. Angio-Cath

    o C. Javid

    o D. Fogarty

160. **What is the best synthetic substitute for stainless steel?**

o A. Surgical silk

o B. Polypropylene

o C. Chromic gut

o D. PTFE

161. **Which of the following microorganisms is used within the biological indicator for ethylene oxide sterilization?**

o A. *Streptococus pneumoniae*

o B. *Pseudomonas aeruginosa*

o C. *Bacillus stearothermophilus*

o D. *Bacillus atrophaeus*

162. **What does the suffix -itis mean?**

o A. Inflammation

o B. Occlusion

o C. Incision

o D. Excision

163. **To prevent peel pack pouches from opening during sterilization, the surgical technologist should:**

o A. Force out air from pouch

o B. Verify correct placement of item inside pouch

o C. Double peel pack all items

o D. Confirm temperature of sterilizer is not too high

164. **Retention bridges are used to:**

o A. Allow for easy removal of sutures

o B. Prevent heavy sutures from cutting into the skin

o C. Keep postoperative drains in place

o D. Designate sutures that are to be removed first

165. **During a CABG procedure, the saphenous vein is sutured to the:**

o A. Superior vena cava

o B. Coronary artery

o C. Subclavian artery

o D. Brachiocephalic artery

166. **Which of the following would be used to remove the lamina during a laminectomy?**

o A. Key elevator

o B. Liston bone cutter

o C. Penfield dissector

o D. Kerrison rongeur

167. What category of instruments are a Hibbs and Hohmann?

    o A. Hemostats

    o B. Retractors

    o C. Bone-holding

    o D. Periosteal elevators

168. Which drain should the surgical technologist have available for insertion into the common bile duct during an exploration?

    o A. Tenckhoff

    o B. Pezzer

    o C. T-tube

    o D. Robinson

169. A padded footboard is used in which surgical position?

    o A. Lithotomy

    o B. Reverse Trendelenburg

    o C. Trendelenburg

    o D. Kraske

170. The inner lining of the gastrointestinal tract is composed of which type of tissue?

    o A. Areolar

    o B. Connective

    o C. Muscle

    o D. Epithelial

171. Which of the following statements is incorrect when double peel packing an item(s) for sterilization?

    o A. Inner peel pack is sterile

    o B. Heavy items should be double peel packed

    o C. Do not bind multiple items together

    o D. Inner peel pack is folded

172. If a surgeon performs a surgical procedure without the patient having signed the consent form, the surgeon can be charged with:

    o A. Battery

    o B. Iatrogenic injury

    o C. Liability

    o D. Negligence

173. Spores are a:

    o A. Type of parasite

    o B. Type of virus

    o C. Form assumed by rickettsia

    o D. Form assumed by bacilli

174. **Which of the following applies to a patient who suffers a burn due to improper placement of the patient return electrode?**

    o A. Unintentional tort
    o B. Res ipsa loquitur
    o C. Intentional infliction
    o D. Doctrine of foreseeability

175. **Which graft material does not require pre-clotting for placement during an abdominal aortic aneurysmectomy?**

    o A. PTFE
    o B. Polyester
    o C. Dacron®
    o D. Fascia lata

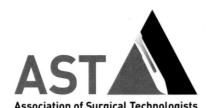
1.	A	31.	B	61.	B	91.	A	121.	B	151.	D
2.	D	32.	A	62.	B	92.	C	122.	B	152.	D
3.	B	33.	B	63.	C	93.	C	123.	B	153.	B
4.	A	34.	C	64.	D	94.	A	124.	C	154.	D
5.	A	35.	A	65.	D	95.	B	125.	D	155.	B
6.	C	36.	A	66.	C	96.	C	126.	C	156.	D
7.	B	37.	C	67.	D	97.	B	127.	D	157.	A
8.	B	38.	B	68.	A	98.	B	128.	C	158.	A
9.	C	39.	C	69.	D	99.	B	129.	C	159.	C
10.	A	40.	C	70.	D	100.	A	130.	D	160.	B
11.	D	41.	B	71.	D	101.	A	131.	C	161.	D
12.	D	42.	C	72.	C	102.	B	132.	B	162.	A
13.	B	43.	B	73.	B	103.	B	133.	D	163.	A
14.	A	44.	C	74.	B	104.	C	134.	A	164.	B
15.	C	45.	D	75.	B	105.	D	135.	B	165.	B
16.	D	46.	D	76.	C	106.	A	136.	B	166.	D
17.	C	47.	A	77.	C	107.	A	137.	A	167.	B
18.	A	48.	B	78.	B	108.	B	138.	D	168.	C
19.	D	49.	D	79.	C	109.	B	139.	D	169.	B
20.	C	50.	C	80.	C	110.	B	140.	B	170.	D
21.	A	51.	A	81.	D	111.	D	141.	D	171.	D
22.	C	52.	C	82.	A	112.	A	142.	A	172.	A
23.	D	53.	C	83.	C	113.	A	143.	D	173.	D
24.	B	54.	C	84.	D	114.	A	144.	B	174.	A
25.	A	55.	D	85.	B	115.	A	145.	C	175.	A
26.	C	56.	A	86.	A	116.	B	146.	B		
27.	B	57.	C	87.	D	117.	B	147.	B		
28.	B	58.	D	88.	D	118.	A	148.	B		
29.	B	59.	D	89.	B	119.	B	149.	B		
30.	A	60.	B	90.	C	120.	D	150.	B		

1. **A.** The Brown-Adson tissue forceps are used during minor procedures to grasp tissue.

2. **D.** The angioscope is used for visualization of the heart and major vessels.

3. **B.** Resident microbes habitually live in the epidermis, deep in the crevices and folds of the skin.

4. **A.** The Stamey procedure involves suspending the fascial attachments of the bladder to the rectus fascia with sutures placed through a Stamey needle.

5. **A.** Sclerotherapy is the injection of sodium chloride, dextrose or saline solution into the small varicosities to destroy the lumen.

6. **C.** There are many anatomical triangles throughout the body to aid the surgeon and surgical team in describing the location of a pathology. A direct hernia presents through Hesselbach's triangle.

7. **B.** The sequence of actions completed by the surgical technologist is remove outer pair of sterile gloves, remove drapes, remove gown and gloves, don pair of non-sterile gloves, assist with immediate postoperative care of the patient, break down the Mayo stand and backtable.

8. **B.** Prior to opening sterile supplies for the first case of the day the OR furniture, equipment, surfaces and lights should be wiped down (also referred to as "damp dusting") with a disinfectant solution.

9. **C.** The autonomic nervous system (ANS) conducts impulses to the cardiac muscles.

10. **A.** Oophor/o is the root word for ovary.

11. **D.** When a vascular anastomosis is being performed, it requires the ability to heal and have a long term, secure anastomosis; therefore, absorbable suture would not be used.

12. **D.** Before the incision is made in the uterus, the bladder is dissected free from the uterus and retracted inferiorly.

13. **B.** Aseptic means without sepsis or no pathogens are present.

14. **A.** The Sims uterine curettes have sharp ends that are graduated in size and used during a D&C to obtain endocervical and endometrial tissue specimens.

15. **C.** Prior to positioning the patient undergoing a posterior lumbar laminectomy, endotracheal intubation is completed.

16. **D.** The Pennington clamp may be used by a surgeon to grasp a hemorrhoid for excision or a small piece of the lung during a segmental resection.

17. **C.** Cholesteatoma is a benign tumor that invades the mastoid cavity and destroys the mastoid air cells and can also damage the ossicles.

18. **A.** The needle holder is clamped approximately one-third of the distance from the swaged end of the needle.

19. **D.** Rigid bronchoscopy is usually performed for the removal of foreign objects from the airway of children.

20. **C.** 96% of the body's mass is made up of oxygen, carbon, hydrogen and nitrogen.

21. **A.** The Bailey rib contractor is positioned over two ribs and tightened to bring them together to facilitate suturing.

22. **C.** The gastrocnemius is the muscle that forms the bulk of the upper calf.

23. **D.** Thrombin should be immediately used when reconstituted with saline or discarded if not used within several hours because it loses potency.

24. **B.** The functions of the small intestine are digestion and absorption.

25. **A.** Teeth are composed of dentin, a calcified connective tissue.

26. **C.** The principles that govern the movement of electrons is the electron theory that serves as the basis for the design of all types of electrical equipment.

27. **B.** To aid in controlling gastric secretions, a vagotomy is performed.

28. **B.** The patient most likely is experiencing an obstructed bowel due to the formation of postoperative adhesions.

29. **B.** The head of the pancreas shares the same arterial supply with the duodenum. Since the Whipple procedure is performed for cancer of the head of the pancreas, the duodenum must be removed.

30. **A.** To facilitate placement of the sutures in the hard palate, the surgeon may use a drill with drill bit.

31. **B.** The biceps brachii flexes and supinates the forearm and covers the anterior portion of the upper arm.

32. **A.** Denial is the first stage of the five stages of grief when the patient doesn't accept what is happening to him/her.

33. **B.** The ureteral catheter stent is implanted to bypass partial or total obstructions of the ureter due to ureteral tumors, calculi or strictures.

34. **C.** Once exposure is completed the repair of a rotator cuff begins by creating a bony trough on the humerus near the tuberosity using a rongeur, curette, curved osteotome or powered burr.

35. **A.** Parietal cells are glands located in the stomach and secrete the digestive juice hydrochloric acid.

36. **A.** Electroencephalography is a recording of the electrical activity of the brain used to help diagnose seizure disorders, brain tumors, epilepsy, and injuries to the brain.

37. **C.** The extremity drape has an opening, called a fenestration, for placing over an extremity.

38. **B.** The vagina is a tubular, fibromuscular organ lined with mucous membrane.

39. **C.** The ultrasonic scalpel (Harmonic scalpel) uses a single-use titanium blade attached to a handpiece and connected to a generator that causes the blade to move by rapid ultrasonic motion to cut and coagulate.

40. **C.** The balloon-tipped Fogarty catheter is inserted through an arteriotomy to facilitate removal of an embolus.

41. **B.** One of the pressure points of the supine position is the elbows; gel pads or foam should be used for protection.

42. **C.** The layers initially incised during a trabeculectomy procedure are the conjunctiva and Tenon's capsule.

43. **B.** The surgical technologist should always anticipate strangulated or incarcerated bowel when preparing for an inguinal herniorraphy and have the bowel instruments in the room in case a bowel resection has to be performed.

44. **C.** The Lukens tube is connected to the suction system of the bronchoscope to collect the specimens.

45. **D.** Steel is the least inert material used as a suture material and is used in the presence of a wound infection.

46. **D.** The Stevens tenotomy scissors are used during delicate procedures, such as eye surgery.

47. **A.** The Sims retractor is used most often in gynecologic surgery.

48. **B.** A strangulated hernia occurs when bowel is trapped within the hernia sac, and the blood supply is compromised.

49. **D.** When using the McBurney's incision for an appendectomy, the first muscle encountered is the external oblique which is bluntly divided in the direction of its fibers.

50. **C.** The broad, uterosacral and cardinal ligaments maintain the position of the uterus.

51. **A.** A transverse colectomy is the excision of the transverse colon; an upper midline or transverse incision is made.

52. **C.** The endometrium is the inner layer of the uterus; the abnormal growth and implantation of the tissue on the outside of the uterus is called endometriosis.

53. **C.** An ultrasound is performed to confirm fluid in the peritoneal cavity.

54. **C.** A fracture table is used to position the patient in the supine position to reduce the fracture.

55. **D.** The lateral kidney position provides optimal exposure to the retroperitoneal area of the flank for a transverse incision.

56. **A.** The correct sequence of instruments when a screw is placed in bone is drill, depth gauge, tap and screw driver; the same sequence is used for placement of all the screws.

57. **C.** When blood or pus from a chest injury is not properly drained from the pleural cavity, it coagulates and forms a fibrin layer over the pleura called empyema. Decortication is dissection of the fibrin.

58. **D.** Succinylcholine is the only depolarizing muscle relaxant in use; it acts rapidly but its effects must be allowed to wear off since there is no reversal agent currently available.

59. **D.** A pantaloon hernia refers to the presence of a direct and indirect hernia.

60. **B.** When placing a patient in the lateral position, the lower leg is flexed and the upper leg is straight with a pillow placed between the legs.

61. **B.** The neuroglia are specialized nerve cells that provide support and protection.

62. **B.** A closed system allows complete rebreathing of expired gases; exhaled carbon dioxide is absorbed by soda lime.

63. **C.** The surgeon is responsible for moving the unsplinted fracture to protect it from further injury when positioning the patient.

64. **D.** Fluoroscopy may be used to identify the exact location of the urinary stone; therefore, the surgical team should wear a lead apron.

65. **D.** The Yankauer is also referred to as the Tonsil suction tip. The angle of the suction tip makes it ideal for pharyngeal suctioning during a tonsillectomy.

66. **C.** Placement of a small pad under the patient's head in the supine position allows the strap muscles to relax and avoids neck strain.

67. **D.** Every time the surgical technologist passes a medication to the surgeon, he/she should verbally provide the name of the drug, strength, and amount.

68. **A.** There are several types of bone holding clamps that vary in size. One type is the Dingman that has a single tooth on the end for grasping the bone.

69. **D.** The Satinsky vena cava clamp, also called the Satinsky partial occlusion clamp, is an atraumatic clamp available in various lengths used during major cardiothoracic procedures such as the CABG.

70. **D.** An absolute requirement of Standard Precautions is the wearing of adequate protective eyewear on all surgical procedures.

71. **D.** Meckel's diverticulum is a congenital diverticulum that presents as a small bulge in the small intestine and can present signs and symptoms that are the same as acute appendicitis.

72. **C.** A double-cuffed tourniquet is used. One cuff is inflated, and if it becomes uncomfortable for the patient, the other cuff is inflated and the first deflated.

73. **B.** A form of liquid medication is an emulsion; the medication is mixed with water and oil and held together by an emulsifier. A common emulsion used in surgery is propofol

74. **B.** The average normal respiration rate for children (1-7 years of age) is 18-30 per minute.

75. **B.** Angiography is the primary diagnostic procedure performed for the evaluation of peripheral vascular disease.

76. **C.** The mesentery is approximated to aid in keeping the intestine in normal anatomical position in order to prevent herniation and maintain the blood supply.

77. **C.** The Association for the Advancement of Medical Instrumentation recommends that instrument sets should not exceed 25 lbs.

78. **B.** The multi-holed ventricular catheter is placed in the lateral ventricle of the brain.

79. **C.** Leiomyomas are a type of uterine fibroid that can cause lower abdominal pain, pelvic congestion, menorrhagia, dysmenorrhea and increased fertility. A myomectomy is a surgical procedure performed to remove the fibroids.

80. **C.** The ureters enter the urinary bladder medially from the posterior aspect.

81. **D.** The pathogen that is most commonly associated with the cause of postoperative SSIs is *Staphylococcus aureus.*

82. **A.** The spleen is the number one organ injured during motor vehicle accidents.

83. **C.** The surgeon's preference card lists the supplies, equipment, instrumentation, suture, dressing materials and surgeon's personal preferences for a procedure.

84. **D.** Non-absorbable sutures become encapsulated during the healing process and remain in the tissues for many years.

85. **B.** Mentoplasty is reconstruction of the chin which can involve placement of a prosthesis.

86. **A.** Phagocytosis is the engulfment of large particles and is sometimes called cell "eating."

87. **D.** The sciatic nerve is a long nerve that extends through the muscles of the thigh, leg, and foot with numerous branches. When a patient is placed in Fowler's (sitting) position, adequate padding must be provided to prevent damage to the nerve.

88. **D.** Hair covers are donned first to decrease the possibility of hair shedding on the scrub suit and decrease microbial shedding.

89. **B.** The vestibulocochlear (VIII) is the cranial nerve that contains special fibers for hearing as well as balance.

90. **C.** Xeroform is a nonpermeable, occlusive dressing made of fine mesh gauze; it is commonly used as the first layer in a three-layer dressing.

91. **A.** Endotoxins cause the overstimulation of coagulating proteins, which causes systemic intravascular clotting that, in turn, results in tissue necrosis.

92. **C.** Materials that allow the flow of free electrons are called conductors and include copper, aluminum, brass and carbon.

93. **C.** Intra-articular refers to 'within a joint;' therefore, the surgeon will be injecting the local anesthetic inside the joint.

94. **A.** Plethysmography is useful in patients with small arterial vessel disease; it records variations in the amount of blood in an extremity.

95. **B.** EtO is the most effective sterilizing agent for items that can be eroded or corroded, because it is heat and/or moisture sensitive.

96. **C.** The mandible articulates with the temporal bone.

97. **B.** In the supine position, crossing the patient's arms across his/her chest causes interference with respirations by tightening the thoracic region and not allowing full expansion of the lungs.

98. **B.** Rubber bands, paper clips or tape should not be used to hold items together inside a peel pack; the binding material prevents the sterilizing agent from making contact.

99. **B.** 98.6–32 = 66.6; 66.6÷1.8 = 37° C

100. **A.** Instruments with multiple parts, such as the Balfour retractor, should be disassembled when breaking down the backtable and Mayo stand.

101. **A.** An example of a short bone are the carpal bones of the wrist; the exception is the pisiform which is a sesamoid bone.

102. **B.** Third intention or delayed primary closure heals by contraction, granulation and connective tissue repair.

103. **B.** The first step in the decontamination process begins at the point of use in the OR. The surgical technologist is responsible for presoaking the instruments in a container of either sterile water, enzymatic or detergent solution.

104. **C.** An enzyme solution is best, since it removes moistened and dried debris without requiring mechanical action.

105. **D.** PTFE is nonabsorbable and should not be used when an infection is present.

106. **A.** Sterile packages can be placed inside a protective plastic wrap/bag called a dust cover to provide additional barrier protection.

107. **A.** The diagonal stripes on the steam autoclave tape and the stripe on the chemical indicator strip should change to black when exposed to the steam sterilization parameters.

108. **B.** The Lowman bone holding clamp, nicknamed "turkey claw," is used for grasping medium-sized bones, such as the radius and ulna to reduce a fracture and hold in place.

109. **B.** The renal vein of the donor kidney is attached to the external iliac vein by an end-to-side anastomosis.

110. **B.** Orchiopexy is performed to treat testicular torsion, position a retracted testicle or undescended testicle.

111. **D.** The incision is made in the inferior posterior portion of the tympanic membrane with a disposable myringotomy knife.

112. **A.** The inner layer of the dressing covers the wound completely and remains in contact. A nonpermeable dressing is a fine mesh gauze that is impregnated with an emulsion; examples are Vaseline® gauze and Xeroform™ gauze.

113. **A.** A straight, curved or angled aneurysm clip is placed across the neck of the aneurysm.

114. **A.** OU (oculus uterque) is the abbreviation for both eyes. Atropine sulfate is a commonly used mydriatic drug that dilates the pupil and is instilled preoperatively for cataract surgery.

115. **A.** The patient's request should be fulfilled; refusal of the request can cause anxiety and irritation in the patient who needs reassurance from the clergy person.

116. **B.** If cultures are not immediately transported to the pathology department, they should be placed in a refrigerator.

117. **B.** A fomite is an inanimate object that is not in itself harmful, but able to harbor pathogenic organisms, thus serving as an agent for transmission of infection.

118. **A.** The patient is placed in the supine position with a bolster placed under the right side to prevent excessive pressure on the inferior vena cava.

119. **B.** The conducting fibers that run from the atrioventricular (AV) node down the inteventricular septum is referred to as the bundle of His.

120. **D.** Items that do not allow the passage of X-rays are referred to as radiopaque. Examples include contrast media and the radiopaque strip on sterile sponges.

121. **B.** At teaching healthcare facilities where surgical technology students complete rotation, CSTs who have an interest in teaching and working with adult learners serve in the preceptor role.

122. **B.** A sterile Doppler probe will be used to identify the superior and inferior epigastric arteries; the superior vessels must be preserved.

123. **B.** Rubber or Silastic items should not be folded, tightly rolled or placed in a mound because steam will either not penetrate or displace the air. The Esmarch bandage should be loosely rolled with a layer of Webril™ in between.

124. **C.** The correct order of the four layers of the colon are mucosa, submucosa, muscularis, serosa.

125. **D.** Dead space is the space caused by separation of wound edges and leads to the accumulation of air or fluid which can then lead to a surgical site infection.

126. **C.** The first step in opening a sterile package is to open the first flap away from the body, side flaps next and last flap toward body.

127. **D.** The patient is positioned supine with the head slightly turned away from the affected side for a unilateral frontotemporal approach.

128. **C.** Ties are loaded onto long-right angle clamps to facilitate placing around vessels.

129. **C.** The pH level of a solution or other liquid such as blood refers to its acidity versus alkalinity levels.

130. **D.** The surgeon usually uses a #11 knife blade to make the initial stab incision for placement of the trocars.

131. **C.** Phagocytic white blood cells engulf and destroy bacteria.

132. **B.** There are several negative body language signals that should be avoided when communicating with patients, patient's family members, peers and the public including tightly folded arms, distancing oneself from patient, frowning, and tapping fingers or foot.

133. **D.** H2 blockers, such as cimetidine, ranitidine and sodium citrate, inhibit hydrochloric acid secretion in the stomach or neutralize stomach acid.

134. **A.** The religious values and standards of Jehovah's Witness should be recognized and upheld by the surgery team including no transfusion of blood. There are other blood replacement products available.

135. **B.** 3:5=9:x; 3/5 = 9/x; 9x5 = 3x; 45=3x; 15=x

136. **B.** The O'Sullivan-O'Connor self-retaining retractor is commonly used during total abdominal hysterectomy.

137. **A.** To facilitate placement of the sutures in the prostatic fossa to control bleeding and reconstruct the bladder outlet, the surgeon may use a Heaney needle holder.

138. **D.** The osteophytes are removed with a Kerrison rongeur.

139. **D.** A subcuticular closure is often used during plastic surgery procedures; the technique minimizes scarring.

140. **B.** The fibula is commonly used to obtain a composite graft to reconstruct the mandible.

141. **D.** When the drill or saw is being used, it produces heat which can char and destroy the bone. A suction irrigator is used by the surgical technologist to prevent heat build-up.

142. **A.** The classic signs of inflammation are pain, heat, redness, swelling and loss of function in reaction to injured tissues.

143. **D.** The Babcock clamp is the primary atraumatic instrument for grasping the appendix during an appendectomy.

144. **B.** The inner layer of the uterus is the endometrium; the outer layer is the perimetrium, and middle layer is the myometrium.

145. **C.** Liquid collodion is a type of chemical dressing that is applied to the wound and dries forming a seal; it is often used for pediatric procedures.

146. **B.** There are certain instances when the initial count and possibly subsequent counts may be omitted. Two examples are emergency cesarean section and ruptured abdominal aortic aneurysm.

147. **B.** When needlestick occurs, the surgical technologist should immediately remove the needle from the sterile field.

148. **B.** The thyroid drape is approximately the same size as a laparotomy drape and has a transverse fenestration.

149. **B.** The cells of Leydig are specialized cells that secrete the male hormone testosterone.

150. **B.** The surgeon usually divides the rectus sheath and muscle with electrosurgery.

151. **D.** The patient skin prep is level of umbilicus to the foot, including the hip region and entire circumference of the leg and entire foot.

152. **D.** The skin prep boundaries are nipple line to symphysis pubis and often extended to midthigh and bilaterally.

153. **B.** Clean scrub attire is worn to protect the patient and surgery staff by limiting the spread of microbes.

154. **D.** Most substances are not absorbed into the blood from the stomach; the absorption takes place in the small intestine. However, some substances that are absorbed from the stomach are water, electrolytes, some drugs and alcohol.

155. **B.** When applying sterile technique, the drape should be removed and a new drape placed.

156. **D.** The TA linear stapling device is best used for dividing the esophagus for removal.

157. **A.** Demyelination can occur when a patient is undergoing radiation therapy and/or chemotherapy for cancer treatment.

158. **A.** A Gigli saw may be used by the surgeon to cut the cranium between the burr holes during a craniotomy.

159. **C.** The Argyle and Javid are two types of shunts used during a carotid endarterectomy.

160. **B.** Polypropylene is the suture material of choice as a substitute for stainless steel when strength and nonreactivity are required, but stainless steel is not appropriate for use in the tissue.

161. **D.** *B. atrophaeus* in spore form is placed within the EtO BI.

162. **A.** The suffix -itis means inflammation such as appendicitis.

163. **A.** As much air as possible should be forced out of the peel pack to prevent bulging and rupture during the sterilization cycle.

164. **B.** Bridges are plastic devices that are placed over the incision like a bridge; retention sutures are brought through holes in the bridge and tied in the middle.

165. **B.** To reestablish blood flow and reoxygenate the heart muscle, the saphenous vein or internal mammary artery is sutured to the coronary artery to bypass the obstruction.

166. **D.** A Kerrison rongeur is used to excise the lamina followed by the pituitary rongeur to remove disk material.

167. **B.** The Hibbs and Hohmann retractors are used in large orthopedic surgical procedures.

168. **C.** The T-tube is used for insertion into the common bile duct to facilitate bile drainage; one arm of the "T" is placed distally, and the other arm placed proximally.

169. **B.** The reverse Trendelenburg (head up) position requires the use of a padded footboard to keep the patient from sliding off the OR table.

170. **D.** The inner lining of the GI tract is composed of epithelium.

171. **D.** The inner peel pack should not be sealed or folded to prevent the entrapment of air during sterilization.

172. **A.** If a surgeon performs surgery without having obtained a signed consent by the patient, the commission of battery has occurred.

173. **D.** Spores are a form assumed by bacilli in order to survive adverse conditions; in this form, they are the most difficult microorganism to be destroyed by methods of sterilization.

174. **A.** Patient burns are usually considered an unintentional tort or, in other words, an error that is reported as an adverse patient incident.

175. **A.** Polytetrafluoroethylene (PTFE) is a non-absorbable flexible material that is used for grafting during an AAA; it does not require preclotting.

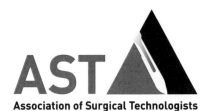
Directions: *Be sure to read each question carefully and select the best answer. You have four hours to complete the test. After finishing the test, review the answers and score your exam.*

In order to pass the CST examination, you must answer 118 questions correctly. If you achieved that score—congratulations! If not, take the time to identify what topics you struggled with and review the appropriate material.

1. **Which cranial nerve is affected by trigeminal neuralgia?**

   o A. I
   o B. V
   o C. VI
   o D. VII

2. **What is used to lubricate the donor site and reduce friction from the dermatome?**

   o A. Bacitracin ointment
   o B. Iodophor solution
   o C. Petrolatum gel
   o D. Mineral oil

3. **Which of the following is an example of proper sterile technique when performing the prep for a split-thickness skin graft?**

   o A. Donor site first
   o B. Recipient site first
   o C. Donor site only
   o D. Recipient site only

4. **What is the recommended range of intra-abdominal pressure in an adult patient when using an insufflator during a laparoscopic procedure?**

   o A. 8–11 mm Hg
   o B. 12–15 mm Hg
   o C. 16–19 mm Hg
   o D. 20–23 mm Hg

5. **Which of these terms refers to the inability to direct both eyes at the same object?**

   o A. Strabismus
   o B. Chalazion
   o C. Glaucoma
   o D. Cataract

6. **What procedure is performed to correct chronic cerebral ischemia?**

   o A.   Rhizotomy

   o B.   Cranioplasty

   o C.   Arteriography

   o D.   Endarterectomy

7. **According to the Rule of Nines, what percentage is assigned to the front and back of the trunk?**

   o A.   27%

   o B.   18%

   o C.   4½%

   o D.   1%

8. **Which term refers to an abnormal increase in the number of cells?**

   o A.   Atrophy

   o B.   Dysplasia

   o C.   Hyperplasia

   o D.   Hypertrophy

9. **A second intention wound heals by:**

   o A.   Granulation

   o B.   Evisceration

   o C.   Primary union

   o D.   Delayed suturing

10. **Intraoperative ventricular arrhythmias are treated with:**

   o A.   Lidocaine

   o B.   Digitoxin

   o C.   Prostigmin

   o D.   Furosemide

11. **How many milliliters equal two (2) ounces?**

   o A.   40

   o B.   50

   o C.   60

   o D.   70

12. **Covering a sterile backtable for later use is:**

   o A.   Permissible for up to one hour before the procedure

   o B.   Permissible in instances of an emergency

   o C.   Not permissible for up to 2 hours before the procedure

   o D.   Not permissible under any circumstances.

13. **In which position would a patient be placed to counteract hypovolemia?**

o A. Left lateral

o B. Right lateral

o C. Trendelenburg

o D. Reverse Trendelenburg

14. **Which of the following types of suture create the least tissue trauma and drag?**

o A. Swaged multifilament

o B. Swaged monofilament

o C. Threaded multifilament

o D. Threaded monofilament

15. **Which organization has legal oversight for the safety of healthcare providers in the work place?**

o A. EPA

o B. CDC

o C. OSHA

o D. NIOSH

16. **Which level of Maslow's Hierarchy of Needs is most applicable to the surgical patient?**

o A. Esteem and prestige

o B. Love and belonging

o C. Safety and security

o D. Physiological and survival

17. **Which of the following would be incorrect technique when removing the sterile gown and gloves?**

o A. Circulator unties gown

o B. Gown removed inside-out

o C. Gloves removed inside-out

o D. Gloves removed first

18. **What type of procedure might require a laparoscopy combination drape?**

o A. Pilonidal cystectomy

o B. Subacromial decompression

o C. Abdominoperineal resection

o D. Femorofemoral bypass

19. **Cell destruction by steam sterilization occurs by:**

o A. Cellular membrane damage

o B. Interrupt cellular division

o C. Altering cellular DNA

o D. Coagulation of protein

20. **Which technique is not acceptable when draping?**

- o A. Hold the drapes 12 inches above patient until over the draping site
- o B. Protect gloved hand by cuffing end of drape over it
- o C. Unfold drape before bringing up to the OR table
- o D. Place drapes on dry area when setting up backtable

21. **A patient's fingernail polish is removed to:**

- o A. Prevent surgical wound infection
- o B. Allow temperature to be recorded
- o C. Prevent ESU exit pathway
- o D. Allow for use of pulse oximeter

22. **What is the purpose of maintaining the air exchange rate at 15—20 times per hour in the OR?**

- o A. Reduce microbial count
- o B. Increase humidity
- o C. Provide comfortable environment
- o D. Decrease static electricity

23. **How many mL of water is necessary to inflate a 5-mL balloon on the Foley indwelling catheter?**

- o A. 5
- o B. 10
- o C. 15
- o D. 20

24. **If an ophthalmologist orders trimming of eyelashes, how is it safely performed?**

- o A. Electric trimmer used on dry lashes
- o B. Electric trimmer used on wet lashes
- o C. Fine scissors without water-soluble gel
- o D. Fine scissors coated with water-soluble gel

25. **What is the correct technique for performing the surgical skin prep?**

- o A. Incision site to periphery using circular motion
- o B. Periphery to incision site using circular motion
- o C. Incision site to periphery using back-and-forth motion
- o D. Periphery to incision site using back-and-forth motion

26. **The laboratory test that determines the ratio of erythrocytes to whole blood is:**

- o A. Reticulocyte count
- o B. Differential count
- o C. Hematocrit
- o D. Hemoglobin

27. **What is the proper procedure to follow when a pack of sponges contains an incorrect number after the patient has entered the OR?**

   o   A.   Record actual number and use
   o   B.   Hand off the sterile field and isolate
   o   C.   Place on sterile backtable and do not use
   o   D.   Remove from the OR

28. **Which of the following types of specimens would not be placed in a preservative solution?**

   o   A.   Colon
   o   B.   Calculi
   o   C.   Tonsils
   o   D.   Uterus

29. **Where should the surgical technologist begin when performing closing counts?**

   o   A.   Backtable
   o   B.   Mayo stand
   o   C.   Off the field
   o   D.   Operative field

30. **Which of the following catheter tips is used in a patient with a urethral stricture?**

   o   A.   Olive
   o   B.   Coude
   o   C.   Whistle
   o   D.   Mushroom

31. **Which type of procedure would require a stent dressing?**

   o   A.   Neck
   o   B.   Inguinal
   o   C.   Extremity
   o   D.   Abdominal

32. **Which of the following is used in order to ensure preservation of the facial nerve during a parotidectomy?**

   o   A.   Monopolar cautery
   o   B.   Nerve stimulator
   o   C.   Microscope
   o   D.   Doppler

33. **Which of the following hemostatic agents is contraindicated for use in the presence of infection?**

   o   A.   Topical thrombin
   o   B.   Oxidized cellulose
   o   C.   Absorbable gelatin
   o   D.   Absorbable collagen

34. During closure of a nephrectomy in the lateral position, the OR table is straightened to facilitate:

o A. Proper circulation

o B. Wound hemostasis

o C. Adequate respirations

o D. Tissue approximation

35. Which of the following must be tested prior to the use of a fiberoptic bronchoscope?

o A. Light source

o B. Laser fiber

o C. Nitrogen level

o D. Magnification lens

36. Excision of a constricted segment of the aorta with reanastomosis is performed to correct:

o A. Patent ductus arteriosus

o B. Coarctation of the aorta

o C. Aortic aneurysm

o D. Transposition of the great vessels

37. For which of the following diagnoses would a patient undergo endoscopic retrograde cholangiopancreatography?

o A. Cholecystitis

o B. Choledocholithiasis

o C. Pancreatitis

o D. Pancreatolithiasis

38. The high ligation of the gonadal veins of the testes performed to reduce venous plexus congestion is a/an:

o A. Spermatocelectomy

o B. Varicocelectomy

o C. Epididymectomy

o D. Vasovasostomy

39. Trauma to which two of the following cranial nerves would result in the loss of smell and vision?

o A. I and II

o B. I and III

o C. II and III

o D. II and IV

40. Which of the following is performed for suspected ectopic pregnancy?

o A. Culdocentesis

o B. Colposcopy

o C. Culdotomy

o D. Colporrhaphy

41. **Which of the following is a procedure for treatment of glaucoma?**

o A. Vitrectomy

o B. Iridectomy

o C. Enucleation

o D. Keratoplasty

42. **What procedure is performed to immobilize the jaw following a mandibular fracture?**

o A. Arch bar application

o B. TMJ osteotomy

o C. LeFort I

o D. LeFort II

43. **Which of the following total arthroplasty procedures would require the postoperative use of an abduction splint?**

o A. Hip

o B. Knee

o C. Ankle

o D. Shoulder

44. **Untreated acute otitis media may result in:**

o A. Tonsillitis

o B. Mastoiditis

o C. Adenoiditis

o D. Ethmoiditis

45. **Which of the following is used intraoperatively to assess vascular patency?**

o A. Positron emission tomography

o B. Magnetic resonance imaging

o C. Computed tomography

o D. Doppler ultrasound

46. The instrument shown below would be used during a:

o A. Parotidectomy

o B. Tonsillectomy

o C. Rhytidectomy

o D. Stapedectomy

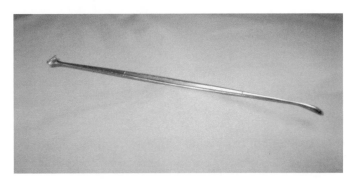

47. Which of the following is the body's primary source of energy?

o A. Carbohydrates

o B. Vitamins

o C. Proteins

o D. Fats

48. What is compressed during rapid-sequence induction and intubation?

o A. Hyoid

o B. Manubrium

o C. Thyroid gland

o D. Cricoid cartilage

49. What term refers to the spread of cancerous cells to other parts of the body?

o A. In-situ

o B. In-vivo

o C. Metastasis

o D. Encapsulation

50. The shared passageway for food and air is the:

o A. Trachea

o B. Larynx

o C. Pharynx

o D. Bronchus

51. The structure that lies along the posterior border of the testis is the:

o A. Prostate

o B. Epididymis

o C. Tunica vaginalis

o D. Ejaculatory duct

52. **The valve between the left atrium and the left ventricle is the:**

o A. Bicuspid

o B. Tricuspid

o C. Aortic semilunar

o D. Pulmonary semilunar

53. **Which characteristic describes an amphiarthrosis?**

o A. Hinge

o B. Immobile

o C. Slightly movable

o D. Freely movable

54. **What is the most abundant ion in the body?**

o A. Calcium

o B. Sodium

o C. Potassium

o D. Magnesium

55. **Which of the following is a method of bacterial survival when environmental conditions are not conducive to growth and viability?**

o A. Conjugation

o B. Transduction

o C. Spore formation

o D. Genetic mutation

56. **What organ detects changes in the level of insulin and releases chemicals to regulate the level of blood glucose?**

o A. Liver

o B. Stomach

o C. Pancreas

o D. Gallbladder

57. **What does the term strike-through mean?**

o A. Rupture of heat seal during sterilization

o B. Failure of biological indicator during sterilization

o C. Perforation of sharp object through sterile wrapper

o D. Soaking of moisture from unsterile to sterile layers

58. **Which of the following monitoring devices would be used within a vessel?**

o A. ECG lead

o B. Swan Ganz

o C. Pulse oximeter

o D. Sphygmomanometer

59. When adding 30 mL of injectable saline to 30 mL of 0.5% Marcaine, what strength does the drug become?

o A. 0.25%

o B. 0.5%

o C. 0.75%

o D. 1.0%

60. What action should be taken if the patient has withdrawn the surgical informed consent prior to surgery?

o A. Transport patient to OR; inform surgeon

o B. Do not transport patient; inform surgeon

o C. Do not transport patient; inform anesthesia provider

o D. Transport patient to OR; inform OR supervisor

61. Confining and containing instruments with bioburden prevents which of the following?

o A. Fomite formation

o B. Personnel injury

o C. Instrument loss

o D. Cross-contamination

62. The unsterile size of the perimeter of a sterile wrap is:

o A. ½ inch

o B. 1 inch

o C. 2 inches

o D. 3 inches

63. A substance that inhibits the growth and reproduction of microbes on living tissue is a/an:

o A. Antiseptic

o B. Disinfectant

o C. Sterilant

o D. Sporicidal

64. What action should be taken by the transporter if a discrepancy occurs in the identification of a patient in the nursing unit?

o A. Try to locate family members to verify patient identity

o B. Transport to OR and inform surgeon of discrepancy

o C. Inform unit clerk of discrepancy and return to OR

o D. Do not transport, inform unit supervisor and OR personnel

65. A patient may be asked to shower at home with an antimicrobial soap before coming to the hospital for surgery to:

o A. Achieve a cumulative antimicrobial effect

o B. Determine if the patient is allergic to the soap

o C. Reduce the amount of time for the pre-op prep

o D. Leave a visible film so the prep borders will show

66. **What are the sequential steps performed prior to entrance into the sterile field?**

o   A.   Gown, glove, scrub

o   B.   Glove, scrub, gown

o   C.   Scrub, glove, gown

o   D.   Scrub, gown, glove

67. **Which area is prepped last when performing the skin prep for a Bartholin's cystectomy?**

o   A.   Anus

o   B.   Mons pubis

o   C.   Vagina

o   D.   Perineum

68. **The sterile surgical technologist should drape a table from:**

o   A.   Side to side

o   B.   Back to front

o   C.   Front to back

o   D.   Open drape, lay it down

69. **Which of the following can be injured if the arm is placed on the arm board greater than 90 degrees?**

o   A.   Brachial plexus

o   B.   Cervical plexus

o   C.   Rotator cuff

o   D.   Acromioclavicular joint

70. **What is the purpose of the third lumen in a three-way indwelling Foley catheter?**

o   A.   Obtain urine specimen

o   B.   Instill irrigation fluids

o   C.   Provide hemostasis

o   D.   Prevent urine reflux

71. **Which of the following enlarges and illuminates the surgical field during cataract procedures?**

o   A.   Fluorescent overhead lights

o   B.   Fiberoptic headlamps

o   C.   Operating microscope

o   D.   Surgical loupes

72. **Small radiopaque surgical patties used during cranial procedures are:**

o   A.   Raytecs

o   B.   Kittners

o   C.   Pledgets

o   D.   Cottonoids

73. **Which of the following hemostatic agents must be applied dry and only handled with dry gloves and instruments?**

o A. Oxycel

o B. Avitene

o C. Gelfoam

o D. Thrombin

74. **Which surgical specialty would utilize a phacoemulsification machine?**

o A. Neurosurgery

o B. Maxillofacial

o C. Ophthalmology

o D. Otorhinolaryngology

75. **Which of the following lasers would be contraindicated for use in the posterior chamber of the eye?**

o A. Argon

o B. Excimer

o C. Ho:YAG

o D. Carbon dioxide

76. **In which structure of the heart are the leads for a permanent pacemaker placed?**

o A. Right ventricle

o B. Left ventricle

o C. Septum

o D. Aorta

77. **For which of the following diagnoses would a patient require pancreaticojejunostomy?**

o A. Gastroschisis

o B. Morbid obesity

o C. Neonatal jaundice

o D. Alcoholic pancreatitis

78. **In which procedure would a Bookwalter retractor be used?**

o A. Cystectomy

o B. Nephrectomy

o C. Retropubic prostatectomy

o D. Transurethral prostatectomy

79. **Which cranial nerve is severed as a last resort treatment of Meniere's disease?**

o A. VII

o B. VIII

o C. IX

o D. X

80. **Brachytherapy is performed to treat:**

o A. Uterine prolapse

o B. Endometriosis

o C. Cervical cancer

o D. Menorrhagia

81. **Which procedure is performed to improve the vision of patients with myopia?**

o A. Radial keratotomy

o B. Scleral buckling

o C. Keratoplasty

o D. Vitrectomy

82. **The facial fracture that involves the complete separation of the maxilla from the cranial base is a/an:**

o A. Orbital floor

o B. Zygomatic

o C. LeFort I

o D. Frontal sinus

83. **What is the name of this retractor?**

o A. Charnley

o B. Bennett

o C. Harrington

o D. Richardson

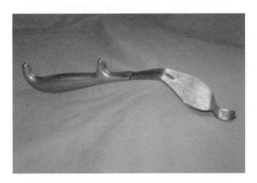

84. **Where is the incision for a Caldwell-Luc procedure made?**

o A. Canine fossa

o B. Frontal sinus

o C. Eyebrow

o D. Tear duct

85. **The device used for real-time intraoperative assessment of blood flow is a/an:**

o A. Caliper

o B. Doppler

o C. Pacemaker

o D. Manometer

86. **The needle holder shown below would be used during a:**

o A. Vaginal hysterectomy

o B. Repair of rotator cuff

o C. Tonsillectomy

o D. Craniotomy

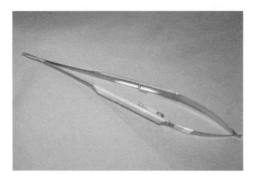

87. **A chemical reaction that provides energy by the breakdown of food is:**

o A. Anabolism

o B. Catabolism

o C. Metabolism

o D. Commensalism

88. **Which structure of the ear is responsible for equilibrium?**

o A. Semicircular canals

o B. Cranial nerve V

o C. Labyrinth

o D. Cochlea

89. **The first step of urine production when fluids and dissolved substances are forced through a membrane by pressure is called:**

o A. Tubular secretion

o B. Tubular reabsorption

o C. Glomerular filtration

o D. Glomerular absorption

90. **The adipose tissue overlying the symphysis is the:**

o A. Labia majora

o B. Mons pubis

o C. Perineum

o D. Vestibule

91. **The cranial nerve that regulates secretion of gastric juice is the:**

o A. III

o B. V

o C. VII

o D. X

92. **Phagocytosis by the white blood cells is an example of which line of defense?**

o A. First

o B. Second

o C. Third

o D. Fourth

93. **When opening a sterile wrapper, the unsterile person should open the first corner:**

o A. Away from self

o B. Toward self

o C. To the right

o D. To the left

94. **Which of the following is the least inert of the synthetic meshes?**

o A. PTFE

o B. Polypropylene

o C. Polyester fiber

o D. Polyglactin 910

95. **What radiopaque contrast medium is used intraoperatively when the patient is allergic to iodine?**

o A. Isovue

o B. Renografin

o C. Methylene blue

o D. Indigo carmine

96. **Which of the following legal terms would apply to a case when a non-English speaking patient signs a surgical informed consent in English, but does not fully understand it?**

o A. Assault and battery

o B. *Res ipsa loquitur*

o C. *Respondeat superior*

o D. Negligence

97. **Which of the following psychosocial factors is important for the surgical team to address for pediatric patients?**

o A. Reliance on others

o B. Postoperative schedule

o C. Separation anxiety

o D. Appearance of scar

98. **What is the surgical technologist's role during the transfer of the patient from the OR bed to the stretcher?**

o A. Completes counts and signs the OR record

o B. Maintains sterility and integrity of backtable

o C. Begins breakdown of sterile setup after drapes removed

o D. Does not remove sterile attire, but aids in patient transfer

99. **When breaking down the sterile field, the surgical technologist should place the grossly contaminated instruments in which of the following?**

o A. Biohazardous bag

o B. Mesh-bottomed flash pan

o C. Basin with sterile saline

o D. Basin with sterile water

100. **How many minutes are unwrapped instruments with no lumens sterilized at 270 degrees F?**

o A. 3

o B. 6

o C. 9

o D. 12

101. **What is the recommended method of hair removal from an operative site?**

o A. Wet shave with disposable razor

o B. Cream depilatory two days pre-op

o C. Clippers with disposable heads

o D. Dry shave with straight razor and tape

102. **Which of the following must be in the chart prior to the patient being taken to the OR per The Joint Commission?**

o A. Incident report

o B. Advance directive

o C. Insurance authorization

o D. History and physical

103. **An identification bracelet is placed on a surgical patient upon admission to the:**

o A. Facility

o B. Nursing unit

o C. Pre-op care unit

o D. Surgery department

104. **To maintain control of the stretcher, the patient should be transported to the OR:**

o A. According to surgeon's orders
o B. Based on patient's request
o C. Head first
o D. Feet first

105. **At what point is it appropriate to lower the leg when draping for a knee arthroscopy?**

o A. After the tourniquet has been inflated
o B. Before the tourniquet has been deflated
o C. After the prep is completed
o D. Before exsanguination

106. **Which structure regulates the amount of light entering the eye?**

o A. Pupil
o B. Iris
o C. Retina
o D. Cornea

107. **A capillary network of blood vessels within the renal cortex that functions as a filter is called the:**

o A. Loop of Henle
o B. Renal papillae
o C. Glomerulus
o D. Nephron

108. **The kidneys are located in the:**

o A. Pelvic cavity
o B. Thoracic cavity
o C. Space of Retzius
o D. Retroperitoneal space

109. **The most abundant extracellular ion necessary for the transmission of impulses is:**

o A. Sodium
o B. Calcium
o C. Chloride
o D. Potassium

110. **The set of teeth that erupt at about 6 months of age and are later replaced are the:**

o A. Secondary dentition
o B. Deciduous teeth
o C. Third molars
o D. Bicuspids

111. **What is a frequently used IV barbiturate for general anesthesia induction?**

o A. Propofol
o B. Ketamine
o C. Thiopental
o D. Lorazepam

112. **Which of the following arteries does not arise directly from the aorta?**

o A. Celiac
o B. Vertebral
o C. Superior mesenteric
o D. Left common carotid

113. **How long must an item be immersed in glutaraldehyde to be sterile?**

o A. 10 minutes
o B. 90 minutes
o C. 6 hours
o D. 10 hours

114. **Which chemical substance causes the immune system to form antibodies?**

o A. Antigens
o B. Interferons
o C. Complements
o D. Immunoglobins

115. **What is a surgical procedure for the treatment of acute otitis media?**

o A. Myringotomy
o B. Stapedectomy
o C. Mastoidectomy
o D. Tympanoplasty

116. **How is the patient positioned on the OR table for a knee arthroscopy?**

o A. Trendelenburg, knee over center break
o B. Lateral, hip over lower break
o C. Supine, knee at lower break
o D. Low lithotomy, body centered

117. **Which of the following instrument sets will be needed when a frontal sinus fracture repair is performed?**

o A. Plastic
o B. Craniotomy
o C. Ophthalmic
o D. Vascular

118. **Which of the following procedures is performed for cervical incompetence?**

o A. Culdocentesis

o B. Colporrhaphy

o C. Wertheim

o D. Shirodkar

119. **What surgical instrument is used to visualize the prostate and remove tissue during a TURP?**

o A. Otis urethrotome

o B. Van Buren sounds

o C. Resectoscope

o D. Ureteroscope

120. **Which of the following facilitates exposure for thyroidectomy?**

o A. Interscapular pillow

o B. Lateral rotation

o C. Mayfield headholder

o D. Reverse Trendelenburg

121. **Which of the following needles would be used for a liver biopsy?**

o A. Stamey

o B. Verres

o C. Tru-Cut

o D. Interstitial

122. **Why is cardioplegia used?**

o A. Inhibit blood vessel spasm

o B. Cause diastolic arrest

o C. Increase force of contraction

o D. Correct acidosis

123. **What is the risk if a tourniquet is inflated for a prolonged period of time?**

o A. Tissue necrosis

o B. Hematoma formation

o C. Hypotension

o D. Tetany

124. **What type of specialty equipment uses liquid nitrogen and is often utilized to repair retinal detachments?**

o A. Nezhat

o B. CUSA

o C. Nerve stimulator

o D. Cryotherapy unit

125. **What is done to the umbilicus during the abdominal skin prep?**

o A. Dabbed with first foam sponge only

o B. Not prepped to prevent contamination

o C. Prepped separately with cotton applicators

o D. Filled with prep solution and left pooled

126. **An axillary role is placed for lateral positioning to:**

o A. Aid venous return

o B. Facilitate respiration

o C. Create good body alignment

o D. Allow access to incision site

127. **Which nerve could be damaged by improperly padded stirrups?**

o A. Tibial

o B. Sciatic

o C. Gluteal

o D. Peroneal

128. **Frozen sections are sent to pathology:**

o A. Immediately without preservative

o B. Immediately with preservative

o C. End of case with preservative

o D. End of case without preservative

129. **Which of the following procedures would be performed with the patient in the lateral position?**

o A. Suprapubic prostatectomy

o B. Vaginal hysterectomy

o C. Nephrectomy

o D. Tonsillectomy

130. **Which heat-resistant, spore-forming Bacillus does the steam sterilization biological indicator contain?**

o A. *S. aureus*

o B. *B. tetani*

o C. *E. coli*

o D. *G. stearothermophilus*

131. **The process by which blood cells are formed is known as:**

o A. Erythropoiesis

o B. Hemopoiesis

o C. Diapedesis

o D. Leukocytosis

132. **The pacemaker of the heart is/are the:**

o A. SA node

o B. AV node

o C. Purkinje fibers

o D. Bundle of His

133. **Thought processes take place in the:**

o A. Midbrain

o B. Cerebellum

o C. Cerebral cortex

o D. Foramen magnum

134. **Kantrex, bacitracin or Ancef mixed with saline for irrigation would do which of the following?**

o A. Minimize vasospasm

o B. Prevent clot formation

o C. Reduce adhesions formation

o D. Inhibit surgical site infection

135. **Which of the following sterilizers operates with condition, exposure, exhaust and dry cycles?**

o A. Gravity air displacement

o B. Prevacuum steam

o C. Hydrogen peroxide

o D. Activated glutaraldehyde

136. **Preoperative bladder drainage prior to a D & C would be performed with which of the following catheters?**

o A. 16 Fr. Foley

o B. 14 Fr. Robinson

o C. 10 Fr. Pezzer

o D. 8 Fr. Malecot

137. **In the OR, HEPA is a type of:**

o A. Air filter

o B. Laminar flow

o C. Suction device

o D. Gas outlet

138. **What precaution is utilized to prevent cardiovascular complications when positioning an anesthetized patient?**

o A. Maintain neutral alignment

o B. Pad bony prominences

o C. Move patient slowly

o D. Uncross legs or ankles

139. **Why is the orientation of the vein graft reversed during a CABG?**

o A. Thickness of tunica intima

o B. Prevent atherosclerosis

o C. Reduce vascular flow

o D. Presence of valves

140. **Which of the following neurosurgical retractors is handheld?**

o A. Greenburg

o B. Cushing

o C. Leyla

o D. Beckman

141. **Which of the following incisions may be used for the repair of a zygomatic fracture?**

o A. Below lower eyelid

o B. Coronal

o C. Angle of the mandible

o D. Preauricular

142. **The principal male hormone produced in the testes is:**

o A. Inhibin

o B. Prolactin

o C. Aldosterone

o D. Testosterone

143. **All of the following statements are true for paper-plastic peel packs, except:**

o A. Felt-tip markers should only be used on the plastic side of pack

o B. Latex tubing should not be used to protect tip of instruments

o C. Staples are an acceptable method of closing peel packs

o D. Inner pack of a double peel-packed item should not be sealed

144. **Following a TURP, a patient may have which of the following placed for bladder irrigation and compression?**

o A. T-tube

o B. 3-way Foley

o C. Robinson

o D. Jackson-Pratt

145. **Which of the following is a correct statement when using the closed-gloving technique?**

o A. Circulator assists with gloving

o B. Hand must not extend beyond cuffs

o C. Fingers of glove are pointed away from elbow

o D. Glove is positioned palm up to facilitate pulling on

146. **What drainage device is preferred for a radical neck dissection?**

o A. T-tube
o B. Penrose
o C. Malecot
o D. Jackson-Pratt

147. **Which arteries are formed by the bifurcation of the abdominal aorta?**

o A. Femoral
o B. Renal
o C. Mesenteric
o D. Iliac

148. **The basic unit of the nervous system is the:**

o A. Neuron
o B. Glial cell
o C. Neurilemma
o D. Schwann cell

149. **The correct sterilization times required to render specific items sterile are initially established by the:**

o A. Healthcare facility policies
o B. Equipment manufacturer
o C. Surgeon's preference
o D. CDC

150. **What procedure involves a series of treatments that result in permanent placement of prosthetic teeth?**

o A. LeFort II
o B. Odontectomy
o C. Orthognathic
o D. Dental implants

151. **In addition to temperature, time and moisture, what other factor determines the outcome of the steam sterilization process?**

o A. Weight
o B. Aeration
o C. Pressure
o D. Concentration

152. **The inner lining of the uterus is the:**

o A. Perineum
o B. Peritoneum
o C. Myometrium
o D. Endometrium

153. Which of the following sterilization processes is most economical?

o A. Gas

o B. Steam

o C. Liquid chemical

o D. Ionizing radiation

154. The basic, living structural and functional unit of the body is known as the:

o A. Organism

o B. Tissue

o C. Organ

o D. Cell

155. The roof of the mouth is formed by the:

o A. Filiform papillae

o B. Palatoglossal arch

o C. Hard and soft palates

o D. Circumvallate papillae

156. In what position would a patient be placed following a tonsillectomy?

o A. Sitting

o B. Lateral

o C. Trendelenburg

o D. Reverse Trendelenburg

157. What classification of drug reduces tissue inflammation?

o A. Steroids

o B. Antibiotics

o C. Antiemetics

o D. Sulfonamides

158. What is the result of adding epinephrine to a local anesthetic?

o A. Prevent clotting

o B. Inhibit infections

o C. Decrease heart rate

o D. Prolong anesthetic effect

159. Which of the following is not a type of sterilizing agent?

o A. Cobalt 60

o B. Boiling water

o C. Steam under pressure

o D. Activated glutaraldehyde

160. **A diagnostic procedure performed for patients with possible prostatic cancer is known as a:**

o A. Needle biopsy

o B. TURP

o C. KUB

o D. Cystostomy

161. **How many hours is the steam biological indicator incubated?**

o A. 4

o B. 6

o C. 12

o D. 24

162. **What agent is used to flush the harvested saphenous vein during a CABG?**

o A. Thrombin

o B. Bacitracin

o C. Heparinized saline

o D. Potassium chloride

163. **In which of the following cases might the surgeon use a Gigli saw?**

o A. Craniotomy

o B. Corpectomy

o C. Cranioplasty

o D. Cordotomy

164. **Low level disinfectants kill most microbes, but typically do not destroy:**

o A. Viruses

o B. Bacteria

o C. Fungi

o D. Spores

165. **Polymethyl methacrylate would most likely be used on which of the following procedures?**

o A. Intramedullary nailing

o B. Total knee arthroplasty

o C. Triple arthrodesis

o D. Percutaneous pinning

166. **Which of the following items should not be sterilized by dry heat?**

o A. Oil

o B. Powder

o C. Linen packs

o D. Petroleum gauze

167. **What is a Verres needle used for during a laparoscopy?**

    o A. Instill CO_2

    o B. Aspirate fluid

    o C. Collect a specimen

    o D. Assist in trocar site closure

168. **Which method uses ultrasonic energy to fragment the lens?**

    o A. Diathermy

    o B. Cryotherapy

    o C. Irrigation/aspiration

    o D. Phacoemulsification

169. **In which of the following procedures would fine hooks of various angles be used?**

    o A. Myringotomy

    o B. Tonsillectomy

    o C. Stapedectomy

    o D. Tympanotomy

170. **Which incisional approach would be used for a splenectomy?**

    o A. Pfannenstiel

    o B. Right subcostal

    o C. Left subcostal

    o D. Supraumbilical

171. **During a strabismus correction, resection has a greater effect on which muscle?**

    o A. Superior rectus

    o B. Inferior rectus

    o C. Medial rectus

    o D. Lateral rectus

172. **What is the best site for obtaining cortical bone graft?**

    o A. Iliac crest

    o B. Ischial spine

    o C. Femoral head

    o D. Symphysis pubis

173. **Which of the following is a non-electrolytic and isotonic solution used during a TURP?**

    o A. Saline

    o B. Distilled water

    o C. Glycine

    o D. Ringer's lactate

174. **The structure that allows the eardrum to vibrate freely and connects the middle ear and the oropharynx is the:**

   o A. External auditory canal
   o B. Eustachian tube
   o C. Semicircular canal
   o D. Internal auditory meatus

175. **Which of the following procedures may require use of a manometer to check CSF pressure?**

   o A. Transphenoidal hypophysectomy
   o B. Intracranial aneurysm clipping
   o C. Posterior fossa decompression
   o D. Ventriculoperitoneal shunt

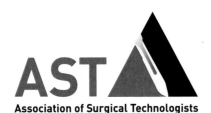

ASSOCIATION OF SURGICAL TECHNOLOGISTS

PRACTICE EXAM #3 ANSWER KEY

1.	B	31.	A	61.	D	91.	D	121.	C	151.	C
2.	D	32.	B	62.	B	92.	B	122.	B	152.	D
3.	A	33.	D	63.	A	93.	A	123.	A	153.	B
4.	B	34.	D	64.	D	94.	C	124.	D	154.	D
5.	A	35.	A	65.	A	95.	B	125.	C	155.	C
6.	D	36.	B	66.	D	96.	A	126.	B	156.	B
7.	B	37.	B	67.	A	97.	C	127.	D	157.	A
8.	C	38.	B	68.	C	98.	B	128.	A	158.	D
9.	A	39.	A	69.	A	99.	D	129.	C	159.	B
10.	A	40.	A	70.	B	100.	A	130.	D	160.	A
11.	C	41.	B	71.	C	101.	C	131.	B	161.	D
12.	D	42.	A	72.	D	102.	D	132.	A	162.	C
13.	C	43.	A	73.	B	103.	A	133.	C	163.	A
14.	B	44.	B	74.	C	104.	D	134.	D	164.	D
15.	C	45.	D	75.	D	105.	A	135.	A	165.	B
16.	D	46.	B	76.	A	106.	B	136.	B	166.	C
17.	D	47.	A	77.	D	107.	C	137.	A	167.	A
18.	C	48.	D	78.	C	108.	D	138.	C	168.	D
19.	D	49.	C	79.	B	109.	A	139.	D	169.	C
20.	C	50.	C	80.	C	110.	B	140.	B	170.	C
21.	D	51.	B	81.	A	111.	C	141.	A	171.	D
22.	A	52.	A	82.	C	112.	B	142.	D	172.	A
23.	B	53.	C	83.	B	113.	D	143.	C	173.	C
24.	D	54.	A	84.	A	114.	A	144.	B	174.	B
25.	A	55.	C	85.	B	115.	A	145.	B	175.	D
26.	C	56.	C	86.	D	116.	C	146.	D		
27.	B	57.	D	87.	B	117.	B	147.	D		
28.	B	58.	B	88.	A	118.	D	148.	A		
29.	D	59.	A	89.	C	119.	C	149.	B		
30.	B	60.	B	90.	B	120.	A	150.	D		

1. **B.** Trigeminal neuralgia arises from the irritation of the fifth cranial nerve.

2. **D.** Sterile mineral oil is used to lubricate the skin at the donor site to reduce friction and provide a smooth surface for the dermatome.

3. **A.** Donor site first is an example of proper sterile technique when performing the skin prep for a split-thickness skin graft.

4. **B.** The intra-abdominal pressure of the carbon dioxide should be maintained between 12-15 mm Hg to avoid damage to the abdomen; however, it should not be allowed to go below 8 mm Hg.

5. **A.** Strabismus is the inability to direct both eyes at the same object due to the lack of coordination of the extraocular muscles.

6. **D.** Indications for a carotid endarterectomy include transient cerebral ischemia, asymptomatic bruits, and chronic cerebral ischemia.

7. **B.** According to the Rule of Nines, the percentage assigned to the front and back of the trunk of the body is 18%.

8. **C.** An abnormal increase in the number of cells due to an increase in the frequency of cell division is known as hyperplasia.

9. **A.** During second intention healing, granulation tissue containing fibroblasts forms in the wound and closes it by contraction with secondary growth of epithelium.

10. **A.** Lidocaine hydrochloride, trade name Xylocaine, is used as an emergency medication during surgery to treat cardiac arrest or ventricular tachycardia or fibrillation.

11. **C.** One fluid ounce equals 30 mL; two ounces equals 60 mL.

12. **D.** Covering a sterile backtable for later use is not permitted, because it is nearly impossible to uncover without contaminating the sterile items on the top of the table; additionally, uncovering the table stirs up dust in the OR.

13. **C.** Hypovolemia is low blood volume. Patients are placed in the Trendelenburg position to increase blood flow to the upper body.

14. **B.** The use of monofilament suture swaged on a needle is best for minimizing tissue trauma and drag.

15. **C.** The Occupational Safety and Health Administration (OSHA) is an organization dedicated to protecting the health of workers by establishing standards that address issues related to safety in the work place.

16. **D.** Physiological and survival is the most applicable to the surgical patient.

17. **D.** The gown is removed first by grasping it near the shoulders and pulling it off. The circulator aids the effort by untying the back of the gown. This action slightly turns the inside of the gloves outward to aid in removing them without touching any patient blood or body fluids that are on the outside of the gloves.

18. **C.** A laparoscopy combination drape is a combination of laparotomy and perineal sheet. It is used for abdominoperineal resection.

19. **D.** The thermal (steam) destruction of microbes is due to the denaturation and coagulation of cellular protein and enzymes.

20. **C.** Drapes are to be carried to the OR table in folded condition. If allowed to unfold, they could drag on the floor contaminating them.

21. **D.** The pulse oximeter cannot properly function with nail polish present. The light beam from the pulse oximeter is focused to travel through the nail and skin of the finger; nail polish changes the color of the light beam causing it to malfunction.

22. **A.** Studies have shown that air exchange in the OR at the rate of 15–20 times per hour helps to reduce the microbial count.

23. **B.** 10 mL of water is necessary to inflate a 5-mL balloon on the Foley indwelling catheter.

24. **D.** Fine scissors coated with water-soluble gel is used for trimming eyelashes.

25. **A.** When performing the patient skin prep, the skin should be scrubbed and painted starting at the incision site using a circular motion.

26. **C.** The percentage or ratio of erythrocytes that is present in the whole blood of the surgical patient is determined by the laboratory test called the hematocrit.

27. **B.** If a sponge pack contains an incorrect number of sponges, the first scrub surgical technologist should hand the sponges to the circulator who will place the sponges in an area of the OR where they will not be thrown away or mixed with other sponges until the end of the procedure and the OR is being cleaned.

28. **B.** Any type of stones, salivary, gallbladder or renal, should be sent dry to pathology. Preservative solutions destroy the stones, making it impossible for pathological examination.

29. **D.** The first scrub should begin at the operative field first and work her/his way backwards—operative field, Mayo stand, backtable, basin, sponge bucket, floor.

30. **B.** Coude is a non-retaining catheter tip to maneuver around an obstruction if a patient has a urethral stricture.

31. **A.** Bolster dressing also referred to as stent dressings are for wounds that are difficult to dress and keep in place, such as the face and neck. The long ends of sutures are tied over the dressing to secure it.

32. **B.** Nerve stimulators create very small electric currents that help to identify and preserve essential facial nerves.

33. **D.** Absorbable collagen is contraindicated in the presence of infection or in areas where blood or other body fluids have pooled.

34. **D.** To achieve proper wound closure, the table must be straightened to bring the tissue of the incision closer together and avoid tension on the suture and tissues.

35. **A.** A fiberoptic light source is the power source for all fiberoptic instruments and equipment and should be tested prior to the use of a fiberoptic bronchoscope.

36. **B.** Coarctation of the aorta can be corrected by excision of a constricted segment of the aorta with reanastomosis.

37. **B.** An endoscopic retrograde cholangiopancreatography (ERCP) is performed to visualize the biliary and pancreatic tract so the patient would have the diagnosis of choledocholithiasis.

38. **B.** The high ligation of the gonadal veins of the testes done to reduce venous plexus congestion is a varicocelectomy.

39. **A.** Surgical trauma to the first and second cranial nerves would cause loss of the sense of smell and sight.

40. **A.** Culdocentensis is a diagnostic procedure performed for suspected ectopic pregnancy, intraperitoneal bleeding or tuboovarian abscess. It involves the aspiration of blood, fluid or pus by needle via the posterior vaginal fornix.

41. **B.** Glaucoma can be surgically treated by performing a goniotomy, iridectomy, or cyclodialysis.

42. **A.** Arch bar application is used to immobilize the jaw following a mandibular fracture.

43. **A.** An abduction splint is used to immobilize and keep in alignment the hip joint following a total hip arthroplasty.

44. **B.** Untreated acute otitis media can lead to mastoiditis.

45. **D.** A Doppler ultrasound device is used intraoperatively to assess vascular patency.

46. **B.** The Hurd dissector and Pillar retractor are used during a tonsillectomy.

47. **A.** The primary source of energy to the body is carbohydrates acquired through the ingestion of carbohydrate-rich foods and liquids.

48. **D.** Sellick's maneuver or cricoid pressure is used to prevent aspiration during induction and ET tube placement.

49. **C.** Metastasis is the spread of cancerous cells to other parts of the body.

50. **C.** The pharynx is a passageway for air and food.

51. **B.** The epididymis is a comma-shaped organ that lies along the posterior border of the testis.

52. **A.** The valve between the left atrium and left ventricle is referred to as either the mitral or bicuspid valve.

53. **C.** An amphiarthrosis refers to a joint that is slightly movable such as the symphysis pubis.

54. **A.** Calcium is the most abundant ion in the body.

55. **C.** Spore formation happens when environmental conditions are not conducive to growth and viability.

56. **C.** The pancreas regulates the concentration of sugar glucose levels in the circulatory system. When the concentration of blood glucose increases, the pancreas senses the change and releases insulin, causing the glucose to move from the blood and be stored in the liver and muscles. When the blood level of glucose is too low, the pancreas releases glucagon that causes stored glucose to be released into the circulatory system.

57. **D.** When moisture soaks through a drape, gown or package, "strike-through" occurs and the item is contaminated.

58. **B.** A Swan Ganz monitoring device is inserted within a branch of the pulmonary artery to measure the central venous pressure, pulmonary artery pressure, pulmonary capillary wedge pressure and cardiac output.

59. **A.** 30 (mL) x .5 (%) = 60 (mL) x X (%)

$$\frac{60 \text{ mL}}{30 \text{mL}} = \frac{.5\%}{X}$$

30 x .5 = 60 x X

15 = 60X

$$\frac{15}{60} = \frac{60X}{60}$$

X = 0.25

60. **B.** If a patient has withdrawn the surgical informed consent prior to surgery, then do not transport patient and inform the surgeon.

61. **D.** Cross-contamination is the contamination of an individual or object upon contact with a contaminated item.

62. **B.** The inside of wrappers is considered sterile except for the one-inch border/perimeter around the outside edge of the wrapper.

63. **A.** Antiseptic agents are used to perform the patient skin prep, as well as used by surgical team members to perform the surgical scrub; the agents are used to "surgically clean" the skin.

64. **D.** Do not transport, inform unit supervisor, and OR personnel if there is a discrepancy in the identification of a patient on the nursing unit.

65. **A.** Studies have shown patients that were asked to shower with antimicrobial soap at home prior to having surgery demonstrate a decrease in the microbial count on the skin.

66. **D.** Before donning the sterile gown and gloves, the sterile members of the OR team must perform the surgical scrub with a chemical antiseptic.

67. **A.** For prepping a Bartholin's cystectomy, the anus is prepped last.

68. **C.** To avoid contamination and reaching over the non-sterile surface when draping a table, the drape should be placed front to back.

69. **A.** If the arm is placed on the arm board at greater than 90 degrees the brachial plexus is at risk for injury.

70. **B.** The third lumen of the three-way indwelling Foley catheter is used for purposes of instilling irrigating fluids into the bladder.

71. **C.** Operating microscope enlarges and illuminates the surgical field.

72. **D.** Cottonoids are small radiopaque surgical patties used during cranial procedures.

73. **B.** Avitene® is a type of collagen material which must be kept dry or it becomes very sticky and difficult to handle.

74. **C.** Phacoemulsification machine uses ultrasonic energy to fragment the lens while it irrigates and aspirates the fragments in ophthalmology surgery.

75. **D.** Carbon dioxide laser would be contraindicated for the use in the posterior chamber of the eye because the laser beam cannot travel through clear fluids.

76. **A.** The endocardial electrode is placed in the right ventricle or atrium.

77. **D.** To relieve pain caused by chronic alcoholic pancreatitis and pseudocysts of the pancreas, a pancreaticojejunostomy may be performed.

78. **C.** Bookwalter retractor may be used for a retropubic prostatectomy.

79. **B.** Méniére's disease is associated with cranial nerve VIII.

80. **C.** Brachytherapy is used in the treatment of cervical cancer.

81. **A.** Radial keratotomy is a procedure performed to improve vision for patients with myopia.

82. **C.** LeFort I fracture is a type of midfacial fracture in which the maxilla is separated from the base of the skull and the upper jaw can be free floating.

83. **B.** Bennett retractors are frequently used in various types of orthopedic procedures.

84. **A.** Caldwell-Luc procedure involves an incision into the canine fossa of the upper jaw.

85. **B.** A Doppler device measures the movement of blood through a vessel using ultrasonic, high-frequency waves.

86. **D.** The Castroviejo needle holder is a type of microsurgical instrument used during delicate cardiothoracic and vascular procedures, and neurosurgery.

87. **B.** The chemical reactions that break down complex organic compounds into simple ones are known as catabolism.

88. **A.** The semicircular canals work to maintain the equilibrium of the body.

89. **C.** The first step in the production of urine is called glomerular filtration.

90. **B.** The elevated adipose tissue over the symphysis is called the mons pubis.

91. **D.** The vagus cranial nerve (X) regulates the secretion of gastric juices.

92. **B.** Phagocytosis by the white blood cells is an example of the body's second line of defense.

93. **A.** When opening a sterile wrapper, the unsterile person should open the corner farthest from the body first. The unsterile person must avoid reaching over a sterile field.

94. **C.** Polyester fiber mesh is one of the least inert of the synthetic meshes.

95. **B.** Renografin is used when a patient is allergic to iodine.

96. **A.** If a non-English speaking patient signs a surgical informed consent in English and does not fully understand it, assault and battery would apply to the situation.

97. **C.** A fear that most pediatric patients experience is anxiety due to impending separation from the parents.

98. **B.** The scrub person should remain sterile and maintain the sterility of the backtable until the patient has left the OR. If any complications should occur in the immediate postoperative period in the OR, the scrub person is prepared to assist.

99. **D.** The dirty instruments should be placed in a basin of water for transport to the decontamination room. Saline will damage the coating on the instruments. The instruments should not be transferred dry to the decontamination room allowing the debris to dry making it difficult to clean.

100. **A.** Instruments that are unwrapped with no lumens can be sterilized at 270 degrees F for 3 minutes.

101. **C.** If a shave is ordered, studies show that the best method is to use clippers with disposable heads to try to prevent cutting or nicking the skin.

102. **D.** Certain information and results of tests should be found in the patient's chart such as lab results, radiology reports, consent form for surgery, previous pathology reports, history and physical reports, allergies, handicaps or other limitations.

103. **A.** Upon admission to the facility, the identification bracelet is placed on the surgical patient.

104. **D.** To allow the individual transporting the patient the ability to control the stretcher and the patient facing in a normal position, the patient is to be transported feet first at all times.

105. **A.** After the tourniquet has been inflated, the leg may be lowered when draping for a knee arthroscopy.

106. **B.** The iris regulates the amount of light entering the eye and assists in obtaining a clear image.

107. **C.** The glomerulus is a capillary network of blood vessels within the renal cortex that functions as a filter.

108. **D.** Since the kidneys are located behind the peritoneal lining of the abdominal cavity, they are retroperitoneal organs.

109. **A.** Sodium is the most abundant extracellular ion necessary for the transmission of impulses.

110. **B.** Deciduous teeth (baby teeth) erupt at about 6 months of age and are lost usually between 6 and 12 years of age.

111. **C.** Thiopental sodium (Pentothal) is a commonly used induction drug.

112. **B.** The celiac, mesenteric, and common carotid arteries arise directly from the aorta; the vertebral arteries arise from the subclavian arteries.

113. **D.** To be considered sterile an item must be completely submerged in glutaraldehyde for 10 hours.

114. **A.** Antigens are chemical substances that react with the body and cause the formation of antibodies.

115. **A.** Myringotomy is an incision into the tympanic membrane in order to suction the infectious fluids and place PE tubes. This is performed for the treatment of chronic acute otitis media.

116. **C.** The patient is placed in the supine position with the knees placed at the lower break of the OR table. The end of the OR table is lowered to facilitate moving the operative leg during the arthroscopy.

117. **B.** A craniotomy approach is often used for frontal sinus repair requiring the use of craniotomy instruments.

118. **D.** The placement of a collar suture at the internal cervical os to prevent spontaneous abortion is called a Shirodkar procedure. Another term for the procedure is cerclage and involves the placement of a polyester (Mersilene®) tape around the internal os and tied.

119. **C.** The resectoscope is a combination of a cutting instrument and an endoscope. The surgeon utilizes a loop electrode that excises the prostatic tissue and the endoscope provides visualization of the prostate.

120. **A.** Several types of devices can be used to hyperextend the neck such as a shoulder roll or interscapular pillow.

121. **C.** A Tru-Cut biopsy needle would be used for obtaining a liver tissue biopsy.

122. **B.** Cardioplegia is used during some open heart procedures to arrest the heart and allow the surgeon the ability to perform the procedure.

123. **A.** Tissue necrosis can occur if the tourniquet is inflated for a prolonged period of time.

124. **D.** The cryotherapy unit uses liquid nitrogen to deliver extreme cold through an insulated probe to the diseased tissue without damaging the adjacent tissues and is often used to repair retinal detachments.

125. **C.** The umbilicus is prepped last or separately since it is considered a contaminated area.

126. **B.** An axillary role is placed for lateral positioning to facilitate respiration.

127. **D.** The peroneal nerve innervates the lateral surface of the lower leg and dorsal surface of the foot. The straps of the stirrups that hold the foot in place if improperly positioned or inadequately padded can cause undue pressure on the nerve causing temporary or permanent damage.

128. **A.** Formalin or normal saline will alter the tissue that is indicated for frozen sections. Therefore, the tissue must be sent in a container with no preservative.

129. **C.** For a nephrectomy, the patient is positioned in the lateral position, non-operative site down.

130. **D.** The biological indicator for steam sterilization contains the *B. stearothermophilus* spore; it is harmless to humans, but is highly resistant to destruction by steam sterilization.

131. **B.** Hemopoiesis is the process by which blood cells are formed.

132. **A.** The sinoatrial (SA) node establishes the rhythm of the heart.

133. **C.** The cerebral cortex, where thought processes occur, is located on the surface of the cerebrum and contains billions of neurons.

134. **D.** Kantrex, bacitracin and Ancef® are antibiotics that are mixed with saline irrigation for purposes of irrigating the surgical wound to prevent a surgical site infection.

135. **A.** Gravity displacement sterilizers have four cycles: condition, exposure, exhaust and dry.

136. **B.** 14 Fr. Robinson should be used prior to a D & C.

137. **A.** HEPA filters are used in the OR due to the ability to remove bacteria as small as 0.5-5 mm.

138. **C.** An anesthetized patient should be moved slowly to allow the cardiovascular system to adjust due to the preoperative and intraoperative drugs the patient has received that affect the system.

139. **D.** The valves within the lumen of the saphenous vein can prevent the flow of blood; therefore, the vein must be reversed when used during a CABG.

140. **B.** Cushing is a handheld neurosurgical retractor.

141. **A.** For zygomaticomaxillary and zygomaticofrontal suture fractures, the incision is placed below the lower eyelid.

142. **D.** Testosterone is the principal male hormone produced in the testes and responsible for sexual characteristics.

143. **C.** Staples must not be used to seal a peel pack; the staples create small holes that create an opening for microbes to enter.

144. **B.** A 3-way Foley may be placed following a TURP.

145. **B.** For closed-gloving, the hand must not extend beyond cuffs.

146. **D.** A Jackson-Pratt drain is preferred for a radical neck dissection when a moderate amount of drainage is expected.

147. **D.** The iliac arteries are formed by the bifurcation of the abdominal aorta.

148. **A.** The basic unit of the nervous system is the neuron.

149. **B.** The sterilization time for an item(s) is established by consulting the manufacturer's recommendations.

150. **D.** Dental implants is a series of treatments that result in a placement of a prosthetic tooth.

151. **C.** The four factors that are important to the steam sterilization process to ensure all microbes are destroyed are temperature, pressure, moisture and air.

152. **D.** The inner layer of the uterus is the endometrium; the outer layer is the perimetrium and the middle layer is the myometrium.

153. **B.** Steam sterilization is the most economical and least expensive method of sterilization.

154. **D.** The basic functional unit of the body that makes up tissues and organs is the cell.

155. **C.** The hard and soft palates form the roof of the mouth.

156. **B.** Postoperatively, a patient is placed in lateral position to prevent aspiration of blood and venous engorgement.

157. **A.** Steroids are a type of drug that reduce tissue inflammation and swelling.

158. **D.** When added to a local anesthetic epinephrine prolongs the anesthetic effect since it is a vasoconstrictor.

159. **B.** The destruction of microbes including spores can be accomplished with steam under pressure, chemical agents such as ethylene oxide, electron bombardment or ultraviolet radiation.

160. **A.** A prostatic needle biopsy is a diagnostic procedure performed when prostatic cancer is suspected.

161. **D.** The steam biological indicator that was put through the steam sterilization process is incubated for 24 hours before the reading is recorded.

162. **C.** The saphenous vein is flushed with heparinized saline to identify branches that may have been missed.

163. **A.** The Gigli saw is used during a craniotomy. It is included in a basic neurologic instrument set.

164. **D.** Low level disinfecting agents kill most bacteria, fungi and viruses, but they are not effective in destroying spores and *M. tuberculosis*.

165. **B.** Polymethyl methacrylate, also known as bone cement, is used for a total joint arthroplasty performed on the knee and hip.

166. **C.** Dry heat is a type of sterilization process used for sterilizing oils, powders and petroleum gauze that will be used in surgery.

167. **A.** The pneumoperitoneum is established by inserting a Verres needle. Tubing from the needle is attached to the insufflator for the instillation of carbon dioxide.

168. **D.** Phacoemulsification uses ultrasonic energy to fragment the lens, while irrigating and aspirating the fragments.

169. **C.** Fine hooks available in varying angles are essential dissecting instruments to perform a stapedectomy.

170. **C.** Incisions commonly used for splenectomy include left subcostal, left paramedian and midline.

171. **D.** When performing a resection for the correction of strabismus, a portion of the lateral rectus muscle is excised, and the two ends reanastomosed.

172. **A.** The iliac crest, the superior portion of the ilium that flares outward, is an excellent source of cancellous and cortical bone for grafting purposes.

173. **C.** Glycine is a non-electrolytic and isotonic solution that is used during a TURP. Since it is non-electrolytic it can be used in conjunction with the resectoscope.

174. **B.** The Eustachian tube connects the middle ear with the nasopharynx of the throat. It ensures that the eardrum vibrates freely when struck by sound waves.

175. **D.** A ventriculoperitoneal shunt is a procedure that may require the use of a manometer to keep track of the intraoperative CSF pressure.

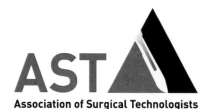
Directions: *Be sure to read each question carefully and select the best answer. You have four hours to complete the test. After finishing the test, review the answers and score your exam.*

In order to pass the CST examination, you must answer 118 questions correctly. If you achieved that score—congratulations! If not, take the time to identify what topics you struggled with and review the appropriate material.

1. **What is used to retract the spermatic cord during an inguinal herniorraphy?**

    o   A.   Skin hook

    o   B.   Penrose drain

    o   C.   Vessel loops

    o   D.   Umbilical tapes

2. **Why is an indwelling Foley catheter placed prior to a hysterectomy?**

    o   A.   Record fluid intake

    o   B.   Avoid injury to bladder

    o   C.   Distend bladder

    o   D.   Demonstrate ureteral patency

3. **Which of the following scissors is the best choice for extending an arterial incision?**

    o   A.   Metzenbaum

    o   B.   Jorgenson

    o   C.   Iris

    o   D.   Potts-Smith

4. **Which of the following is used to stain the cervix for a Schiller's test?**

    o   A.   Lugol's solution

    o   B.   Indigo carmine

    o   C.   Methylene blue

    o   D.   Acetic acid

5. **Which of the following arises from the left ventricle of the heart?**

    o   A.   Ascending aorta

    o   B.   Pulmonary vein

    o   C.   Descending aorta

    o   D.   Pulmonary artery

6.   **What method is used to confirm that items have been exposed to the sterilization process, but sterility is not guaranteed?**

o   A.   Mechanical

o   B.   Biological

o   C.   Chemical

o   D.   Bowie-Dick

7.   **Why would the hair of a patient undergoing craniotomy be bagged, labeled and saved?**

o   A.   To donate to cancer patients

o   B.   In case of need for future genetic testing

o   C.   It is patient property

o   D.   Prevent post-op surgical site infection

8.   **When preparing a double basin for sterilization, the:**

o   A.   Basins should be separated by a porous, absorbent towel

o   B.   Sponges should be placed in the top basin

o   C.   Wrapped package should be laid flat on the shelf of the sterilizing cart

o   D.   Bottom basin should contain a residual of distilled water

9.   **Which structure, during a total hip arthroplasty, requires intramedullary reaming prior to placement of a prosthesis?**

o   A.   Femoral canal

o   B.   Tibial plateau

o   C.   Acetabular fossa

o   D.   Greater trochanter

10.   **Which of the following is the least restrictive form of credentialing?**

o   A.   Certification

o   B.   Licensure

o   C.   Registration

o   D.   Accreditation

11.   **What drug classification is Demerol®?**

o   A.   Dilator

o   B.   Analgesic

o   C.   Sedative

o   D.   Vasoconstrictor

12.   **What should be transported to the PACU with a patient who underwent a thyroidectomy?**

o   A.   Tracheotomy tray

o   B.   Clean stent dressing

o   C.   Extra Penrose drain

o   D.   Antiembolic stockings

13. **What is the chemical abbreviation for sodium chloride?**

   o A. Fe
   o B. Hg
   o C. NaCl
   o D. H20

14. **Which organelle is responsible for packaging of proteins?**

   o A. Golgi complex
   o B. Mitochondria
   o C. Nucleus
   o D. Ribosome

15. **Which procedure would utilize the instrument shown below?**

   o A. D&C
   o B. Hemorrhoidectomy
   o C. Gastrostomy
   o D. TURP

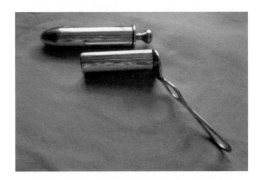

16. **What types of treatment does a patient authorize when signing a general consent form?**

   o A. Only for receiving general anesthesia
   o B. Invasive surgical procedures
   o C. Receiving experimental drugs
   o D. All routine treatments or procedures

17. **Which medication can be used as a topical jelly during cystoscopy procedures?**

   o A. Bupivacaine
   o B. Xylocaine
   o C. Sensorcaine
   o D. Procaine

18. **Which of the following is a primary postoperative complication of carotid endarterectomy?**

   o A. Failure of graft
   o B. Pulmonary embolus
   o C. Pneumonia
   o D. Stroke

19. **During which procedure would the instrument shown below be used?**

   o A. D&C
   o B. TAH
   o C. MMK
   o D. LAVH

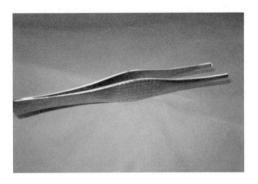

20. **When is it acceptable to open surgical dressing sponges?**

   o A. After first count
   o B. After skin incision
   o C. After final count
   o D. After closure of cavity

21. **What is the correct procedure to follow when a sterilized rigid instrument container is opened and condensation is observed?**

   o A. Don't use; return to Sterile Processing Department
   o B. Let container air dry before use
   o C. Dry out with a sterile towel before using
   o D. Use it; water droplets are sterile

22. **Which method of sterilization requires an aeration cycle?**

   o A. Ionizing radiation
   o B. EtO
   o C. Peracetic acid
   o D. Hydrogen peroxide plasma

23. **Elevated IOP in a glaucoma patient is a result of excess:**

   o A. Vitreous humor
   o B. Aqueous humor
   o C. CSF
   o D. RBC

24. **Where should the grounding pad be placed on a patient undergoing a laparoscopic cholecystectomy who has a right hip prosthesis?**

o A. Left anterior thigh

o B. Right posterior thigh

o C. Lower back

o D. Upper abdomen

25. **The instrument below is used during a:**

o A. Tuboplasty

o B. Vaginal hysterectomy

o C. Laparoscopy

o D. Simple vulvectomy

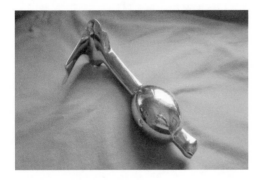

26. **The Trendelenburg position is often used for surgery on the:**

o A. Head and neck

o B. Lower abdomen and pelvis

o C. Lower back and hips

o D. Knee or thigh

27. **The large artery that arises from the left side of the aortic arch and descends into the arm is the:**

o A. Brachiocephalic

o B. Coronary

o C. Subclavian

o D. Axillary

28. **Lesions in which part of the brain may affect balance and coordination?**

o A. Limbic System

o B. Cerebral Cortex

o C. Cerebellum

o D. Medulla

29.   **Which of the following utilizes the process of cavitation?**

o A. Washer-sterilizer
o B. Ultrasonic cleaner
o C. Washer-decontaminator
o D. Steam sterilizer

30.   **Which of the following is the name for a dorsally angulated fracture of the distal radius?**

o A. Smith's
o B. Pott's
o C. Colles'
o D. Bennett's

31.   **During which procedure would the instrument shown below be used?**

o A. Pancreatectomy
o B. Gastrectomy
o C. Splenectomy
o D. Cholecystectomy

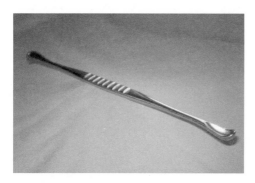

32.   **Which ligament is transected during surgery for De Quervain's disease?**

o A. Dorsal carpal
o B. Adductor pollicis
o C. Transverse carpal
o D. Extensor retinaculum

33.   **In order to minimize mucosal irritation during urinary catheterization, the tip of the catheter is dipped in which of the following?**

o A. Vaseline
o B. K-Y Jelly
o C. Chlorhexidine
o D. Sterile saline

34. **How often is a medication prescribed as QID to be taken per day?**

o A. 4 times

o B. 2 times

o C. 3 times

o D. 1 time

35. **What type of external dressing would be used to eliminate dead space?**

o A. Immobilizing

o B. Bulky

o C. Packing

o D. Pressure

36. **In the prone position, patients are placed on chest rolls to prevent:**

o A. Decubitis ulcers

o B. Lumbar strain

o C. Compromised ventilation

o D. Foot drop

37. **Which of the following positions would be used for an LAVH?**

o A. Lateral

o B. Prone

o C. Sitting

o D. Lithotomy

38. **A left subcostal incision would be used to expose the:**

o A. Descending colon

o B. Spleen

o C. Ovary

o D. Gallbladder

39. **Intraoperatively, lidocaine with epinephrine may be contraindicated in patients who are:**

o A. Immunocompromised

o B. Hypertensive

o C. Dehydrated

o D. Diabetic

40. **What approach is used for the removal of a small acoustic neuroma that is located in the internal auditory canal?**

o A. Suboccipital

o B. Middle fossa

o C. Translabyrinthine

o D. Posterior fossa

41. **Which of the following must be obtained from a patient undergoing surgical procedures, fertility treatments, chemotherapy or experimental treatment?**

o A. General written consent

o B. Special implied consent

o C. Special written consent

o D. General implied consent

42. **What drug is used to treat hypotension and shock?**

o A. Pronestyl

o B. Inderal

o C. Dantrolene

o D. Levophed

43. **The agent used to expand blood plasma volume is:**

o A. Diprivan

o B. Duramorph

o C. Demerol®

o D. Dextran

44. **What does the term chole/ refer to?**

o A. Chyme

o B. Bile

o C. Spleen

o D. Intestine

45. **When preparing instruments for sterilization, all the following are completed with the exception of:**

o A. Maintaining the ringed instruments in an open position

o B. Placing heavy instruments on the bottom of the tray

o C. Placing the instruments in a mesh-bottom tray

o D. Lining the tray with a nonwoven disposable wrapper

46. **Which of the following is an initial incision for abdominoplasty?**

o A. Periumbilical

o B. Upper paramedian

o C. Low transverse

o D. Midline

47. **When performing a rhinoplasty, the exostosis in the nose is removed with a:**

o A. Chisel

o B. Rongeur

o C. Scissors

o D. Saw

48. **Which type of sterilization requires the use of the Bowie-Dick test?**

   o A. Plasma
   o B. Prevacuum steam
   o C. EtO
   o D. Steris®

49. **What is the first federal act to establish patient privacy standards?**

   o A. Health Insurance Portability and Accountability Act
   o B. Patient Protection and Affordable Care Act
   o C. Patient Care Partnership
   o D. Safe Medical Device Act

50. **What should the surgical technologist wear when transporting a patient with tuberculosis from PACU to the isolation patient room?**

   o A. Hair cover
   o B. Surgical mask
   o C. No additional precautions necessary
   o D. Respirator

51. **How is the informed consent signed if a patient is illiterate?**

   o A. Two physicans sign consent
   o B. Surgeon signs consent
   o C. Verbal consent of patient
   o D. Patient marks an 'x'

52. **Which of the following agents should not be used to disinfect endoscopes?**

   o A. Distilled water
   o B. Glutaraldehyde
   o C. Enzymatic solution
   o D. Isopropyl alcohol

53. **Which of the following is used to expose the meatus during urethral catheterization?**

   o A. Cottonball
   o B. Sponge stick
   o C. Non-dominant hand
   o D. Dominant hand

54. **Which of the following is the second phase of wound healing?**

   o A. Proliferation
   o B. Maturation
   o C. Contraction
   o D. Lag

55. **What muscle is commonly used for TRAM reconstruction in a mammoplasty?**

   o A. Latissimus dorsi

   o B. Transverse abdominis

   o C. Internal oblique

   o D. Rectus abdominis

56. **The patient is never positioned until the:**

   o A. Surgical technologist is scrubbed

   o B. Surgeon gives permission

   o C. Circulator has finished all preparatory duties

   o D. Anesthesia provider gives permission

57. **What term refers to cell "drinking"?**

   o A. Osmosis

   o B. Phagocytosis

   o C. Pinocytosis

   o D. Filtration

58. **What does hypertension mean?**

   o A. High blood pressure

   o B. Normal blood pressure

   o C. No blood pressure

   o D. Low blood pressure

59. **Which type of fire extinguisher should be available when using a laser?**

   o A. Water

   o B. Carbon dioxide

   o C. Halon

   o D. Dry chemical

60. **What is the major side effect of thrombolytics?**

   o A. Infection

   o B. Hemorrhage

   o C. Nausea

   o D. Clotting

61. **If a sterile glove becomes contaminated during a procedure, what action should the surgical technologist take?**

   o A. Surgical technologist pulls off glove covering hand with gown cuff; regloves using closed technique

   o B. Circulator pulls off glove covering hand with gown cuff; surgical technologist regloves using closed technique

   o C. Circulator pulls off glove; surgical technologist is regloved by another sterile team member

   o D. Surgical technologist pulls off glove; regloves using open technique

62. **What type of suture technique is used to invert the stump of the appendix during an appendectomy?**

   o A. Purse-string
   o B. Continuous
   o C. Horizontal
   o D. Interrupted

63. **Which of the following is the proper procedure for removing a laparotomy drape?**

   o A. Circulator holds dressing in place and removes drape
   o B. ST holds dressing in place; rolls drape one side to other
   o C. Circulator holds dressing in place; ST rolls drape head to feet
   o D. Surgical technologist (ST) holds dressing in place; rolls drape head to feet

64. **Gerota's fascia is located:**

   o A. Around the kidney
   o B. Within the kidney
   o C. Within the bladder
   o D. Around the bladder

65. **What activity can aggravate the symptoms of trigeminal neuralgia?**

   o A. Typing
   o B. Walking
   o C. Chewing
   o D. Sitting

66. **What is the purpose of maintaining 20% to 60% relative humidity in the OR?**

   o A. Eliminate microbial count
   o B. Provide comfortable environment
   o C. Decrease static electricity
   o D. Reduce room temperature

67. **What surgical instrument is used to thread the drilled hole for the screw during an ORIF?**

   o A. Tap
   o B. Depth gauge
   o C. Osteotome
   o D. Drill bit

68. **Which of the following pathology would be treated by transphenoidal hypophysectomy procedure?**

   o A. Pituitary neoplasm
   o B. Trigeminal neuralgia
   o C. Carotid stenosis
   o D. Communicating hydrocephalus

69. **The muscles that cause strabismus are the:**

o A. Orbicularis oculi

o B. Ciliary

o C. Tarsal plates

o D. Extrinsic

70. **What is the minimum required number of people to transfer a patient from the OR table to the stretcher?**

o A. 6

o B. 5

o C. 4

o D. 3

71. **When used as a skin prep, which of the following should be allowed to thoroughly dry if electrocautery will be used?**

o A. Aqueous solutions

o B. Hexacholorophene

o C. Alcohol and tinctures

o D. Iodophor solutions

72. **Healthcare-acquired infections (HAI) are most commonly associated with which of the following?**

o A. Prolonged bed rest

o B. Use of urinary catheters

o C. Surgical site contamination

o D. Prescribed antibiotic therapy

73. **What is the technical term for robotic arms?**

o A. Manipulator

o B. Telechir

o C. Articulated

o D. Resolution

74. **In which of the following procedures would the surgeon check for anastomotic leaks by injecting air into the rectum, looking for bubbles in the fluid-filled peritoneal cavity?**

o A. Low anterior resection

o B. Nissen fundoplication

o C. Subtotal gastrectomy

o D. Roux-en-Y anastomosis

75. **What are varicosities of the rectum and anus?**

o A. Hemorrhoids

o B. Polyps

o C. Fissures

o D. Sinuses

76. **Vitamins A, D, E and K are absorbed in the:**

o A. Stomach

o B. Intestine

o C. Pancreas

o D. Liver

77. **The preoperative exsanguination of an extremity prior to inflating a tourniquet is accomplished with:**

o A. Webril®

o B. Green towel

o C. Esmarch

o D. Kling

78. **Which of the following vessels is harvested for use during a CABG?**

o A. Azygous vein

o B. Internal mammary artery

o C. Popliteal vein

o D. Left axillary artery

79. **Which of the following retractors would be used to retract the muscles during a hip pinning?**

o A. Harrington

o B. Charnley

o C. Bennett

o D. Richardson

80. **The surgical reanastomosis of the vas deferens is called a:**

o A. Vasovasostomy

o B. Spermatocelectomy

o C. Cystostomy

o D. Varicocelectomy

81. **Which type of laser is used to remove polymethyl methacrylate from a cemented joint implant during a revision arthroplasty?**

o A. Excimer

o B. Argon

o C. Carbon dioxide

o D. Ho:YAG

82. **Sound waves travel through the external auditory canal and strike the:**

o A. Tympanic membrane

o B. Auricle

o C. Oval window

o D. Ossicle

83. **In large abdominal wounds that require frequent dressing changes, which of the following will minimize the skin break-down?**

   o A.   Steri-Strips™

   o B.   Petrolatum gauze

   o C.   Liquid collodion

   o D.   Montgomery straps

84. **Which of the following positioning devices would be used for an LAVH?**

   o A.   Padded footboard

   o B.   Mayfield headrest

   o C.   Allen stirrups

   o D.   Kidney brace

85. **The term mentoplasty refers to surgery of the:**

   o A.   Lip

   o B.   Eyelid

   o C.   Palate

   o D.   Chin

86. **Which of the following situations could cause a patient's signature on a surgical informed consent to be challenged in court?**

   o A.   Patient is of legal age

   o B.   Patient advised of alternative treatments

   o C.   Patient is emancipated minor

   o D.   Patient received preoperative medications

87. **What is the importance of humidity when using EtO sterilization?**

   o A.   Remove chlorofluorocarbons

   o B.   Hydrate spores and bacteria

   o C.   Reduce flammability of gas

   o D.   Prevent instruments from drying

88. **What is the purpose of polymethyl methacrylate during a cranioplasty?**

   o A.   Reducing vascular spasm

   o B.   Filling cranial defects

   o C.   Adhesive skin closure

   o D.   Subarachnoid space dye

89. **The appropriate location when placing the grounding pad is over a:**

   o A.   Keloid scar

   o B.   Bony prominence

   o C.   Metal prosthesis

   o D.   Fleshy area

90. **Which catheter is used for an angioplasty?**

o A. Gruntzig

o B. Robinson

o C. Fogarty

o D. Swan-Ganz

91. **A hernia that presents through Hesselbach's triangle is a/an:**

o A. Pantaloon

o B. Direct

o C. Hypogastric

o D. Indirect

92. **The medial malleolus is part of which bone?**

o A. Tibia

o B. Talus

o C. Calcaneous

o D. Fibula

93. **What is performed prior to implantation of a Dacron® knit polyester graft?**

o A. Soak in thrombin

o B. Preclotting

o C. Heparinization

o D. Immerse in antibiotics

94. **Which structure articulates with the head of the femur?**

o A. Ilium

o B. Pubis

o C. Acetabulum

o D. Ischium

95. **An abnormal bending backward of the uterus is called:**

o A. Cephalic version

o B. Anteversion

o C. Retroperitoneal

o D. Retroflexion

96. **What type of clip is a Raney?**

o A. Scalp

o B. Nerve

o C. Aneurysm

o D. Vessel

97. **The ciliary body is part of which layer of the eye?**

    o A. Lens
    o B. Fibrous
    o C. Nervous
    o D. Vascular

98. **Which of these drugs is a miotic?**

    o A. Tropicamide
    o B. Atropine
    o C. Pilocarpine
    o D. Phenylephrine

99. **Which of the following is a violation of Standard Precautions during postoperative case management ?**

    o A. Sterile gloves removed one layer at a time
    o B. Linen items not thrown into hamper
    o C. Use of bags with biohazard symbol
    o D. Retrieve reusable trocar from sharps container

100. **Which type of monitoring equipment is a noninvasive assessment of oxygen saturation of arterial blood?**

    o A. Electrocardiogram
    o B. Bispectral Index™
    o C. Pulse oximetry
    o D. Capnography

101. **How are femoral shaft fractures in an adult repaired?**

    o A. Hemiarthroplasty
    o B. Kirschner wires
    o C. Closed reduction
    o D. Intramedullary nailing

102. **Which of the following instruments would be used to dilate the male urethra?**

    o A. Pratt
    o B. Bakes
    o C. Van Buren
    o D. Hegar

103. **To determine the process for preparing surgical instruments for use on tissue and within a body cavity, they are classified as:**

    o A. Critical
    o B. Semicritical
    o C. Controlled
    o D. Noncritical

104. **The Harrington retractor allows for gentle elevation of which anatomical structure?**

    o   A.   Stomach
    o   B.   Heart
    o   C.   Liver
    o   D.   Bladder

105. **What is the term for the division of a reproductive cell into two cells with chromosome cells?**

    o   A.   Binary fission
    o   B.   Mitosis
    o   C.   Meiosis
    o   D.   Spontaneous generation

106. **What does the term dys- mean?**

    o   A.   Proximal
    o   B.   Distal
    o   C.   Difficult
    o   D.   Easy

107. **After the patient is extubated, which device is often used to maintain the airway around the relaxed tongue?**

    o   A.   Laryngoscope
    o   B.   Oropharyngeal airway
    o   C.   Stylet
    o   D.   Laryngeal mask airway

108. **Which of the following accelerates the coagulation cascade?**

    o   A.   Papaverine
    o   B.   Epinephrine
    o   C.   Topical thrombin
    o   D.   IV Heparin

109. **Which breast procedure describes a mastectomy?**

    o   A.   Reduction
    o   B.   Surgical removal
    o   C.   Incisional biopsy
    o   D.   Augmentation

110. **What is done to the common bile duct during a choledochojejunostomy?**

    o   A.   Excised
    o   B.   Visualized
    o   C.   Anastomosed
    o   D.   Bypassed

111. **In which of the following procedures would a tourniquet be unnecessary?**

o A. Hip arthroplasty
o B. Knee arthroplasty
o C. Ankle fracture
o D. ORIF radius

112. **Which of the following anatomical sites would be prepped last when performing a skin prep for a colostomy reversal procedure?**

o A. Suprapubic area
o B. Stoma
o C. Umbilicus
o D. Lateral borders

113. **What surgical procedure is performed to relieve pressure on the median nerve?**

o A. Endoscopic carpal tunnel release
o B. Ulnar nerve transposition
o C. Metacarpophalangeal joint replacement
o D. External fixation of radius

114. **What is the proper procedure for turning the sterile gown?**

o A. Circulator removes tag from gown; surgical technologist turns
o B. Hand tag to circulator; surgical technologist and circulator turn
o C. Hand tag to circulator; circulator moves around gown
o D. Surgical technologist holds tag and turns self

115. **What does the term 'os' mean?**

o A. Bone
o B. Opening
o C. Occlusion
o D. Right

116. **Which of the following is not a function of the trachea?**

o A. Carry air to and from the lungs
o B. Amplify speech
o C. Filter secretions and particulates
o D. Humidify inspired air

117. **Which condition is characterized by the sudden onset of floating spots before the eyes?**

o A. Scleral tumor
o B. Retinal detachment
o C. Vitreous hemorrhage
o D. Epiretinal membrane

118. **One of the most effective germicidals for cold sterilization is:**

o A. 2% glutaraldehyde

o B. Alcohol

o C. Hexachlorophene

o D. Betadine

119. **From which laminectomy instrument would intervertebral disc fragments be cleaned?**

o A. Penfield

o B. Langenbeck

o C. Pituitary

o D. Taylor

120. **What type of suture is used for vascular reanastomosis?**

o A. Absorbable multifilament

o B. Nonabsorbable monofilament

o C. Nonabsorbable multifilament

o D. Absorbable monofilament

121. **What is the name of the suction tip?**

o A. Baron

o B. Poole

o C. Frazier

o D. Antrum

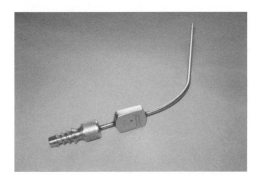

122. **What molecule is broken down when body cells require energy?**

o A. ATP

o B. RNA

o C. DNA

o D. ADP

123. **Which of the following represents a saddle joint?**

o A. Radius and carpals

o B. Thumb and trapezium

o C. Femur and hip

o D. Ulna and radius

124. **During an EtO sterilization cycle, humidity is maintained at:**

o A. 50-90%

o B. 80-100%

o C. 20-80%

o D. 10-25%

125. **An emergency drug given to stabilize ventricular fibrillation is:**

o A. Anectine

o B. Isoproterenol

o C. Vasopressin

o D. Nitroglycerine

126. **Creating a positive-pressure air supply for each OR will:**

o A. Prevent fires during laser surgery

o B. Maintain a stable relative humidity

o C. Minimize airborne bacteria entering room

o D. Reduce external noise and conversations

127. **Which is an acceptable antiseptic solution for a skin prep?**

o A. Povidone-Iodine

o B. Lugol's solution

o C. Hydrogen peroxide

o D. Activated glutaraldehyde

128. **During a total hip arthroplasty, which instrument is used after intramedullary reaming to reshape the proximal femoral canal?**

o A. Rongeur

o B. Curette

o C. Brush

o D. Rasp

129. **Which of the following assesses the electrical activity of the nervous system?**

o A. Spirometry

o B. Electroencephalogram

o C. Peripheral nerve stimulator

o D. Electrocardiogram

130. **The functional unit of the kidney responsible for removing waste and regulating fluid is the:**

o A. Cortex

o B. Renal pelvis

o C. Medulla

o D. Nephron

131. **Which of the following is an intermediate-level disinfectant?**

o A. Isopropyl alcohol

o B. Glutaraldehyde

o C. Peracetic acid

o D. Hydrogen peroxide

132. **Which vein of an infant patient is a central venous catheter inserted?**

o A. Internal jugular

o B. Saphenous

o C. Subclavian

o D. External jugular

133. **After the patient leaves the OR, the reusable items should be taken to the decontamination room:**

o A. By covering instrument tray with bag and carry

o B. Carried in a basin soaking in enzymatic solution

o C. On the shelf of the sterilization cart

o D. Inside a closed case cart

134. **A clamp used for occluding a peripheral vessel is:**

o A. Duval

o B. Allen

o C. Kocher

o D. DeBakey

135. **During a total hip arthroplasty, which type of device prevents polymethyl methacrylate from filling the medullary canal distal to the prosthesis?**

o A. Stem

o B. Restrictor

o C. Brush

o D. Wick

136. **Which of the following is proper technique when applying a grounding pad?**

o A. Avoid placing pad on buttocks

o B. Apply pad before patient is positioned

o C. Apply gel to pad

o D. Reuse pad that is repositioned

137. **Which of the following sutures are packaged in alcohol to maintain pliability?**

o A. Synthetic absorbable

o B. Natural absorbable

o C. Synthetic non-absorbable

o D. Natural non-absorbable

138. **What procedure should be followed for securing consent for surgery for an unconscious patient requiring emergency surgery whose family members or guardian cannot be contacted?**

o A. Chief of Surgery waives consent

o B. Surgeon and Risk Manager sign consent

o C. Two consulting physicians agree

o D. Obtain telephone court order

139. **What gynecologic procedure includes removal of the reproductive organs, bladder and rectum?**

o A. Posterior colporrhaphy

o B. Total hysterectomy

o C. Abdominoperineal resection

o D. Pelvic exenteration

140. **Isopropyl alcohol is bactericidal, which means it:**

o A. Inhibits the growth of bacteria

o B. Sterilizes surfaces

o C. Destroys spores

o D. Kills bacteria

141. **Use of a one-step applicator with little or no pressure on skin would be indicated in which of the following conditions?**

o A. Pleural effusion

o B. Herniated lumbar disc

o C. Abdominal aortic aneurysm

o D. Cholecystitis with cholelithiasis

142. **A postoperative anesthesia complication when extubating a patient is:**

o A. Allergic reaction

o B. Laryngospasm

o C. Hemorrhage

o D. Malignant hyperthermia

143. **The process by which glucose is stored as glycogen is:**

o A. Glucolysis

o B. Glycolysis

o C. Glycogenesis

o D. Gluconeogenesis

144. **The large, leaf-shaped laryngeal cartilage that acts as a "trap door" over the larynx is the:**

o A. Thyroid

o B. Cricoid

o C. Oropharynx

o D. Epiglottis

145. **Use of Van Buren sounds might be necessary for urethral catheterization in patients with which of the following?**

o A. Ureteral calculi

o B. Urethral calculi

o C. Ureteral stricture

o D. Urethral stricture

146. **The four fluid-filled spaces of the brain are:**

o A. Fissures

o B. Auricles

o C. Ventricles

o D. Sulci

147. **For which surgical procedure would bupivicaine with epinephrine be contraindicated?**

o A. Subacromial decompression

o B. Total joint arthroplasty

o C. Knee arthroscopy

o D. Trigger finger release

148. **What term describes an individual who harbors a pathogen but displays no signs or symptoms?**

o A. Fomite

o B. Carrier

o C. Vector

o D. Reservoir

149. **Which of the following procedures is performed before completing an ileal conduit?**

o A. Ureterolithotomy

o B. Prostatectomy

o C. Cystectomy

o D. Ileostomy

150. **Which of the following is the recommended postoperative handling of reusable instruments used on a patient with Creutzfeldt-Jakob disease?**

o A. Place in biohazard bag and destroy

o B. Flash sterilize and transport to central sterile supply

o C. Decontaminate in OR

o D. Transport in case cart to decontamination room

151. **In what anatomical structure would a T-tube most likely be placed?**

o A. Urethra

o B. Ureter

o C. Common bile duct

o D. Lacrimal duct

152. **What type of procedure is performed to treat tumors of the pituitary gland?**

o A. Ventriculoscopy

o B. Craniotomy

o C. Endoscopic microdecompression

o D. Transphenoidal hypophysectomy

153. **Which of the following would be an inappropriate manner for the handling of surgical specimens?**

o A. Permission is given by surgeon to hand specimen off sterile field

o B. Stones and teeth are placed in container without preservative

o C. Cultures are sent to pathology immediately

o D. Frozen sections are sent to pathology on a Raytec sponge

154. **Which of the following instruments would be used during a suprapubic prostatectomy?**

o A. Wertheim pedicle clamp

o B. Iglesias resectoscope

o C. Bladder retractor

o D. Stamey needle

155. **A tumescent solution is used in which of the following procedures?**

o A. Breast augmentation

o B. Scar revision

o C. Collagen injection

o D. Suction lipectomy

156. **Which of the following is a type of non-retaining catheter?**

o A. Foley

o B. Malecot

o C. Whistle

o D. Pezzer

157. **The walls of the vagina are lined with:**

o A. Peritoneum

o B. Serosa

o C. Mucosa

o D. Fascia

158. **Which drug counteracts metabolic acidosis?**

o A. Atropine sulfate

o B. Lidocaine

o C. Sodium bicarbonate

o D. Meperdine

159. **Which of the following wound classifications would be assigned to a compound fracture?**

o A. Clean

o B. Contaminated

o C. Clean-contaminated

o D. Dirty

160. **What type of dye is used intravenously to verify patency of the fallopian tubes during a pelvic procedure?**

o A. Methylene blue

o B. Isovue

o C. Renografin

o D. Gentian violet

161. **Pneumoperitoneum is utilized during a laparoscopy to do which of the following?**

o A. Illuminate cavity

o B. Prevent embolism

o C. Create safe working space

o D. Reduce blood pressure

162. **What is the required pressure for a steam sterilizer set at a temperature of 250°F?**

o A. 24 - 26

o B. 21 - 23

o C. 18 - 20

o D. 15 - 17

163. **What is the most commonly used thermal method of hemostasis in cranial neurosurgery?**

o A. Cryosurgery

o B. Bipolar electrosurgery

o C. Monopolar electrocautery

o D. Hypothermia

164. **A wrapped instrument set that will be run in the steam prevacuum sterilizer at 270° must be sterilized for a minimum of:**

o A. 6 minutes

o B. 2 minutes

o C. 8 minutes

o D. 4 minutes

165. **A patient that has sudden onset of shortness of breath in the PACU may indicate:**

o A. Hypotension

o B. Pulmonary embolism

o C. Air embolism

o D. Asthma attack

166. **Which of the following sutures is a nonabsorbable monofilament frequently used in vascular procedures?**

o A. Polypropylene

o B. Polydiaxonone

o C. Poliglecaprone 25

o D. Polyglactine 910

167. **Which of the following defines anaerobic?**

o A. Without nitrogen

o B. Without oxygen

o C. With nitrogen

o D. With oxygen

168. **Which nerve in the lower leg must be protected from pressure when placing the patient in the lithotomy position?**

o A. Lateral plantar

o B. Biceps femoris

o C. Ulnar

o D. Peroneal

169. **Exophthalmos due to Grave's disease is associated with which gland?**

o A. Parotid

o B. Thyroid

o C. Pituitary

o D. Thymus

170. **Where should the Foley indwelling catheter drainage bag be positioned after insertion of the catheter?**

o A. Above the level of the bladder

o B. Level of the bladder

o C. Lower than the level of the bladder

o D. Position not important

171. **The sutures of the adult skull are examples of:**

o A. Synarthroses

o B. Synchondroses

o C. Syndesmoses

o D. Symphyses

172. **A ventilation system that provides a unidirectional positive-pressure air flow at a high air exchange rate in the OR is:**

o A. Central air

o B. Filtered air conditioning

o C. Conventional air system

o D. Laminar air flow

173. **Catabolism of fats produces:**

o A. Ketone bodies

o B. Glycogen

o C. Amino acids

o D. Bile

174. **What is the principal reason for performing a preoperative skin prep?**

o A. Provide a visible demarcation of prepped borders

o B. Degrease the skin so that incise drapes will adhere

o C. Sterilize the skin to prevent surgical site infection

o D. Remove transient flora and reduce resident flora

175. **What is the part of the brain that is responsible for controlling the body temperature?**

o A. Cerebellum

o B. Pons

o C. Cerebrum

o D. Hypothalamus

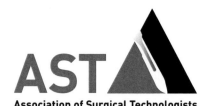

1.	B	31.	D	61.	C	91.	B	121.	C	151.	C
2.	B	32.	A	62.	A	92.	A	122.	A	152.	D
3.	D	33.	B	63.	D	93.	B	123.	B	153.	D
4.	A	34.	A	64.	A	94.	C	124.	C	154.	C
5.	A	35.	D	65.	C	95.	D	125.	B	155.	D
6.	C	36.	C	66.	C	96.	A	126.	C	156.	C
7.	C	37.	D	67.	A	97.	D	127.	A	157.	C
8.	A	38.	B	68.	A	98.	C	128.	D	158.	C
9.	A	39.	B	69.	D	99.	D	129.	B	159.	B
10.	C	40.	B	70.	C	100.	C	130.	D	160.	A
11.	B	41.	C	71.	C	101.	D	131.	A	161.	C
12.	A	42.	D	72.	B	102.	C	132.	D	162.	D
13.	C	43.	D	73.	A	103.	A	133.	D	163.	B
14.	A	44.	B	74.	A	104.	C	134.	D	164.	D
15.	B	45.	D	75.	A	105.	C	135.	B	165.	B
16.	D	46.	C	76.	B	106.	C	136.	A	166.	A
17.	B	47.	A	77.	C	107.	B	137.	B	167.	B
18.	D	48.	B	78.	B	108.	C	138.	C	168.	D
19.	B	49.	A	79.	C	109.	B	139.	D	169.	B
20.	C	50.	D	80.	A	110.	C	140.	D	170.	C
21.	A	51.	D	81.	C	111.	A	141.	C	171.	A
22.	B	52.	D	82.	A	112.	B	142.	B	172.	D
23.	B	53.	C	83.	D	113.	A	143.	C	173.	A
24.	A	54.	A	84.	C	114.	C	144.	D	174.	D
25.	B	55.	D	85.	D	115.	B	145.	D	175.	D
26.	B	56.	D	86.	D	116.	B	146.	C		
27.	C	57.	C	87.	B	117.	B	147.	D		
28.	C	58.	A	88.	B	118.	A	148.	B		
29.	B	59.	C	89.	D	119.	C	149.	C		
30.	C	60.	B	90.	C	120.	B	150.	A		

1. **B.** A ¼" or ½" Penrose drain is used to gently retract the spermatic cord; it should be placed in saline prior to handing to the surgeon.

2. **B.** To decompress the bladder and prevent injury to the organ during a hysterectomy, an indwelling Foley catheter is preoperatively inserted into the patient.

3. **D.** Potts-Smith scissors are available in various angles which allow for inserting into the incision made with the knife blade and extending.

4. **A.** The Schiller test involves staining the cervix with Lugol solution. The glycogen in the cervical epithelium takes up the iodine and abnormal tissues that have little to no glycogen do not stain brown, therefore indicating areas of tissue that should be biopsied.

5. **A.** The portion of the aorta that passes upward behind the pulmonary trunk as it emerges from the left ventricle is called the ascending aorta.

6. **C.** Chemical indicators such as autoclave tape are impregnated with a dye that changes color when exposed to the sterilization process.

7. **C.** The hair is the patient's property. He/she may want to have it formed into a wig, require it for religious reasons, or it may be a memento.

8. **A.** A porous, absorbent towel should be placed between nested basins to absorb condensate, aid in air removal and allow for penetration of steam.

9. **A.** The femoral canal requires intramedullary reaming prior to placement of prosthesis during a total hip arthroplasty.

10. **C.** Registration involves a formal process where qualified individuals are listed in a registry.

11. **B.** Meperidine hydrochloride (Demerol®) is an analgesic.

12. **A.** A tracheotomy tray should be transported with the patient to the PACU and ward room due to the postoperative risks of inflammation and hemorrhage.

13. **C.** The symbol for sodium chloride is NaCl.

14. **A.** The Golgi complex, a group of organelles, processes, sorts, packages, and delivers proteins to the plasma membrane, lysosomes, and secretory vesicles.

15. **B.** The Hirschmann anoscope is one of several types of retractors used to expose the rectal canal during a hemorrhoidectomy.

16. **D.** When a patient signs a general consent form, the patient is agreeing to all routine treatments or procedures.

17. **B.** Lidocaine (Xylocaine) jelly may be put into the urethra as a topical anesthesia for a cystoscopy.

18. **D.** The primary postoperative complication of carotid endarterectomy is stroke; the patient's neurological status must be closely monitored.

19. **B.** The Ferris-Smith tissue forceps is a heavy-duty instrument with teeth that are ideal for use during a total abdominal hysterectomy.

20. **C.** Surgical dressing sponges are opened after the wound is closed, and the final count was performed.

21. **A.** The container must be considered contaminated, removed from the OR, and returned to the sterile processing department.

22. **B.** The aeration cycle is necessary to remove the toxic EtO from the sterile packages and items.

23. **B.** Intraocular pressure is produced chiefly by the aqueous humor.

24. **A.** During a laparoscopic cholecystectomy of a patient who has a right hip prosthesis, the grounding pad should be positioned on the left anterior thigh. This prevents electric current from traveling through the metal and causing a patient burn.

25. **B.** The Auvard weighted vaginal speculum is placed with the blade along the posterior vaginal wall to provide exposure.

26. **B.** The Trendelenburg position allows displacement of the abdominopelvic organs to aid in visualization of the operative site.

27. **C.** The subclavian artery arises from the left side of the aortic arch and descends into the arm.

28. **C.** The cerebellum is at the base of the brain and is responsible for balance and coordination.

29. **B.** The ultrasonic cleaner uses the process of cavitation to dislodge minute particles of soil and debris from surgical instruments.

30. **C.** Colles' fracture is the name for a dorsally angulated fracture and is usually repaired by closed reduction with the use of the C-arm and casting.

31. **D.** The Ferguson gallstone scoop can be used to remove gallstones during a cholecystectomy.

32. **A.** De Quervain's is caused by inflammation of the tendons in the first dorsal compartment of the wrist. The dorsal carpal ligament is cut to release the tendons.

33. **B.** K-Y jelly is used to lubricate the catheter tip to aid in insertion and minimize mucosal irritation.

34. **A.** QID is an abbreviation meaning 4 times per day.

35. **D.** A pressure dressing is a type of three-layer dressing used to eliminate dead space.

36. **C.** Prone position places pressure on the thorax and abdomen making it difficult to breathe; chest rolls are placed to slightly elevate the patient's upper torso to facilitate ventilation.

37. **D.** For an LAVH, the patient is placed in the lithotomy position.

38. **B.** The spleen is located in the left upper quadrant and a left subcostal incision is used for exposure.

39. **B.** Lidocaine with epinephrine is contraindicated in patients who are hypertensive since epinephrine increases the blood pressure.

40. **B.** The middle fossa approach provides good extradural exposure for small tumors.

41. **C.** A special written consent must be obtained from a patient undergoing surgical procedures, fertility treatments, chemotherapy, or experimental treatment.

42. **D.** Levarterenol (Levophed®) is used to treat hypotension and shock.

43. **D.** Dextran is a plasma volume expander that acts by drawing fluid from tissues, thus decreasing blood viscosity.

44. **B.** Chole is a combining form meaning bile.

45. **D.** A nonwoven disposable wrapper should not be used to line the bottom of the tray since the water-repellent wrapper would cause condensate to collect.

46. **C.** The skin incision for an abdominoplasty is a low transverse.

47. **A.** Two surgical instruments commonly used to remove the midline hump in the nose are chisel or rasp.

48. **B.** The Bowie-Dick test is used for prevacuum sterilizers to confirm there is no air entrapment occurring.

49. **A.** HIPAA took effect in 2003; it is the first federal legislation to establish privacy standards for patients.

50. **D.** The CDC and NIOSH recommend the use of a respirator when caring for a TB patient.

51. **D.** When a patient is illiterate, but understands the verbal explanation, he/she marks the informed consent with an 'x.'

52. **D.** Isopropyl alcohol should not be used to clean endoscopes because it breaks down the cement.

53. **C.** The non-dominant hand should be used to expose the meatus, and the dominant hand to insert the catheter.

54. **A.** Phase 2 of wound healing is proliferation which begins approximately on the third postoperative day.

55. **D.** The use of the transverse rectus abdominis musculocutaneous (TRAM) flap is a type of pedicle flap reconstruction in which the tissue is transferred but remains attached to its blood supply.

56. **D.** The anesthetized patient is not moved until permission is given by the anesthesia provider.

57. **C.** In pinocytosis, "cell drinking," the engulfed material is a tiny droplet of extracellular fluid rather than a solid.

58. **A.** Hypertension is a term for high blood pressure.

59. **C.** The halon fire extinguisher is recommended because of its low toxicity and residue is not produced.

60. **B.** The major side effect of thrombolytics is hemorrhage.

61. **C.** The surgical technologist should step away from the sterile field, circulator grasps glove and pulls off leaving hand exposed; he/she is regloved by another member of the sterile team.

62. **A.** The stump of the appendix is inverted into the colon and a circular purse-string suture is placed to maintain the inverted stump.

63. **D.** The proper technique for removing a drape is for the ST to hold the dressing in place while rolling the drape from head to feet, and disposing in the waste receptacle.

64. **A.** Gerota's fascia surrounds the kidney to serve as a cushion.

65. **C.** Trigeminal neuralgia is a condition characterized by severe pain in the face and is paroxysmal. Chewing usually aggravates the symptoms.

66. **C.** Humidity level is kept between 20-60% to prevent static electricity.

67. **A.** Once the hole for a screw has been drilled, the tap is used to pre-place threads within the hole to aid with insertion of the screws.

68. **A.** Transphenoidal hypophysectomy is the procedure of choice for pituitary tumors.

69. **D.** The 6 extrinsic muscles work together to move the eye in various directions; strabismus is due to problems with coordinated eye muscle movement.

70. **C.** The minimum number of people is 4 - anesthesia provider at the head, person at the foot, one person on the far side of the OR table, other person far side of the stretcher.

71. **C.** Alcohol and solutions with alcohol should be allowed to thoroughly dry to prevent the flammable fumes from collecting under the sterile drapes and possibly igniting when electrocautery is used.

72. **B.** HAI are often acquired through the use of indwelling catheters such as the Foley catheter.

73. **A.** The technical term for the robotic arms is manipulator.

74. **A.** Before the surgical wound is closed, the lumen of the bowel is insufflated to check for air leaks from the anastomosis.

75. **A.** Hemorrhoids are thrombosed veins located internally within the rectum and externally at the anus.

76. **B.** Vitamins A, D, E and K are absorbed in the small intestine.

77. **C.** The extremity is elevated and wrapping is distal to proximal with an Esmarch or Ace bandage; once exsanguinated the tourniquet is inflated.

78. **B.** The internal mammary artery or saphenous vein is anastomosed to the affected coronary artery during a CABG.

79. **C.** Bennett retractors are frequently used to retract the muscles during a hip pinning due to the angle of the head of the retractor.

80. **A.** A vasovasostomy is performed for the reanastomosis of the vas deferens.

81. **C.** The carbon dioxide laser is used to vaporize polymethyl methacrylate to aid in the removal of the prosthesis.

82. **A.** Sound waves collect in the auricle and pass on to strike the tympanic membrane.

83. **D.** Montgomery straps are utilized for surgical wounds that require frequent dressing changes. They consist of two sections, the first has an adhesive side that sticks to the skin and a nonadhesive side with strings that are tied over the intermediate dressing layer and can be untied to perform the dressing change.

84. **C.** Allen stirrups, which aid in placing the patient in low lithotomy position, are used for the LAVH procedure.

85. **D.** Mentoplasty is the medical term that refers to plastic surgery of the chin.

86. **D.** If the patient received preoperative medications prior to signing the surgical informed consent, this can be challenged in court.

87. **B.** Moisture hydrates bacteria and spores to reduce their resistance to the gas.

88. **B.** Polymethyl methacrylate is an alloplastic material used to repair cranial defects caused by accidents, tumors, and other trauma.

89. **D.** The pad should be applied to a fleshy area, preferably over a clean and dry muscle mass.

90. **C.** Fogarty catheter is used when performing an angioplasty.

91. **B.** Direct hernia is a type of inguinal hernia that presents within Hesselbach's triangle.

92. **A.** The medial malleolus is part of the tibia.

93. **B.** Due to the porosity of the material that allows blood to seep through, Dacron® knit polyester grafts require preclotting.

94. **C.** The structure that serves as the socket for the head of the femur is the acetabulum, which is formed by the ilium, ischium and pubis.

95. **D.** The ligaments that maintain the position of the uterus are flexible enough to allow the uterus to become malpositioned; retroflexion is a harmless malposition.

96. **A.** The Raney scalp clip is applied to the edges of the incised scalp to control bleeding during cranial procedures.

97. **D.** The ciliary body is located in the anterior portion of the vascular tunic.

98. **C.** Miotics are pupil-constricting agents and pilocarpine hydrochloride is a common miotic used for this purpose.

99. **D.** No item should ever be retrieved from the sharps container to avoid a sharps accident.

100. **C.** Pulse oximetry is the noninvasive assessment of the oxygen level of the arterial blood using a light absorption technique.

101. **D.** Femoral shaft fractures in adults are repaired with either compression plating or intramedullary nailing.

102. **C.** Van Buren is a type of male urethral dilator that is available in diameters that increase in size.

103. **A.** Surgical instruments and other items that will come into contact with the patient's tissues and/or be used within a body cavity are categorized as critical and must be sterile.

104. **C.** A Harrington retractor is a large, deep retractor and allows for gentle retraction of the liver.

105. **C.** The division of a reproductive cell into two cells with 23 chromosomes each is called meiosis.

106. **C.** Dys- is a prefix meaning difficult.

107. **B.** Upon extubation, the ET is usually replaced with an oropharyngeal airway to lift the tongue forward or nasal airway to lift the soft palate from the back of the oropharynx.

108. **C.** Topical thrombin aids in speeding up the coagulation cascade.

109. **B.** Mastectomy means removal of the breast.

110. **C.** Choledochojejunostomy is an anastomosis between the common bile duct and jejunum to reestablish flow of bile.

111. **A.** In a hip arthroplasty, a tourniquet would be unnecessary.

112. **B.** When prepping for a colostomy reversal procedure, the stoma site is prepped last since it is considered contaminated.

113. **A.** A carpal tunnel release involves surgically releasing the transverse carpal ligament to relieve pressure on the median nerve.

114. **C.** The surgical technologist hands the tag to the circulator who moves around to the left side to prevent the surgical technologist from spinning and posssibly contaminating the gown.

115. **B.** An opening or mouth is an 'os.'

116. **B.** The trachea does not assist in ampliflying speech.

117. **B.** The sudden onset of the appearance of floating spots before the eyes is one of the initial symptoms of a retinal detachment.

118. **A.** Glutaraldehyde is an agent that is used for disinfection and sterilization purposes.

119. **C.** Pituitary rongeur, bone drill and nerve hook are all commonly used during a lumbar laminectomy.

120. **B.** Nonabsorbable monofilament suture is used for vascular reanastomosis.

121. **C.** The Frazier suction tip is useful for small incisions and pediatric procedures.

122. **A.** ATP provides energy for various cellular activities in living systems.

123. **B.** An example of a saddle joint is the joint between the trapezium of the carpus and metacarpal of the thumb.

124. **C.** Humidity is maintained at 20-80% within the EtO sterilizer to hydrate the bacteria and spores.

125. **B.** Isoproterenol hydrochloride (Isuprel) is used to treat ventricular fibrillation that occurs during surgery.

126. **C.** To prevent contamination of the air in the OR from air outside the room, pressure in the OR should be positive.

127. **A.** Povidone-Iodine (commercial name Betadine) is an ideal agent to use for the patient skin prep; however, a patient can be allergic to the solution.

128. **D.** The instrument used after intramedullary reaming is a series of rasps from small to large size.

129. **B.** Electroencephalogram is a display and recording of the electrical activity of the brain through the placement of electrodes on the scalp.

130. **D.** The unit of the kidney responsible for removing waste and regulating fluid is the nephron.

131. **A.** Isopropyl alcohol is tuberculocidal, bactericidal, virucidal and fungicidal, but not sporidical.

132. **D.** In neonates and infants, a cutdown approach to the external jugular is preferred for insertion of a central venous catheter.

133. **D.** To prevent cross contamination and airborne microbes, instruments are placed within a closed case cart to transport.

134. **D.** There are several type of DeBakey clamps and the DeBakey peripheral vascular clamp is angled with smooth serrations making it ideal for clamping blood vessels without damaging the tissue.

135. **B.** The cement restrictor is placed at the end of the reamed femoral canal prior to injecting the bone cement to prevent it from entering the medullary canal.

136. **A.** Placing the pad on the buttocks should be avoided since uneven and incomplete contact with the skin will most likely occur.

137. **B.** Natural absorbable sutures are packaged in an alcohol-water based solution to maintain their pliability.

138. **C.** When an unconscious patient requires emergency surgery and the family members or guardian cannot be contacted, two consulting physicians must agree that the surgery is needed.

139. **D.** Pelvic exenteration, a radical pelvic procedure, performed for highly invasive, persistent carcinoma is only performed if it offers the possibility of a cure.

140. **D.** Bacter/i refers to bacteria and -cidal means kill/destroy.

141. **C.** To prevent rupturing the delicate aneurysm, very little pressure should be placed on the abdomen and the prep should be gently performed.

142. **B.** When the patient is extubated, laryngospasm can occur due to irritation and/or inflammation of the airway by the endotracheal tube.

143. **C.** If glucose is not required for ATP production at once, it is mixed with other molecules of glucose to form glycogen, which is then stored in the liver and skeletal muscle fibers, referred to as glycogenesis.

144. **D.** The epiglottis is a large, leaf-shaped piece of cartilage that moves freely over the larynx.

145. **D.** In the presence of a urethral stricture, the use of a Van Buren dilator may be necessary prior to inserting the catheter.

146. **C.** The ventricles are four fluid-filled spaces located in the brain.

147. **D.** Trigger finger release is the procedure that bupivacaine with epinephrine would be contraindicated.

148. **B.** Someone who carries a pathogen without manifesting symptoms is called a carrier.

149. **C.** When the entire bladder is removed (cystectomy), a urinary bladder diversion procedure is required. Ileal conduit is the standard procedure performed after a cystectomy.

150. **A.** The recommendation by the WHO is to place the instruments in an impervious container, place in biohazard bag, label "possible CJD" and destroy the instruments.

151. **C.** The T-tube, due to its configurations, is best used for placement in the common bile duct for drainage of the biliary system.

152. **D.** The pituitary gland is accessed through an incision in the upper gum or nasal cavity and the sphenoid sinus is incised to reach the pituitary gland.

153. **D.** A counted sponge, such as a raytec sponge, must never be used for passing off and transporting a specimen.

154. **C.** A bladder retractor is often used to aid in visualization of the interior of the bladder during the procedure.

155. **D.** A tumescent solution is used in the suction lipectomy procedure.

156. **C.** The Whistle is a type of non-retaining catheter used to obtain urine specimen or decompress the bladder.

157. **C.** The vagina is a tubular, fibromuscular organ lined with mucous membrane.

158. **C.** Sodium bicarbonate is used to correct metabolic acidosis during cardiac arrest.

159. **B.** Compound or open fracture would have a wound classification as contaminated.

160. **A.** Methylene blue is used intravenously to verify patency of the fallopian tubes.

161. **C.** Pneumoperitoneum is established to provide a working space in the abdomen and allow the intestines to fall away from the anterior of the abdominal cavity to prevent perforation by the trocars upon insertion.

162. **D.** The pressure for a steam sterilizer set at 250°F must be 15–17 with a minimum exposure of 15 minutes.

163. **B.** Bipolar electrosurgery, cottonoid strips, and bone wax are all methods of hemostasis commonly used in neurosurgery.

164. **D.** A wrapped instrument set placed in a steam prevacuum sterilizer at 270° F must be exposed to that temperature for a minimum of 4 minutes.

165. **B.** Pulmonary embolism is a primary cause of death intra-and postoperatively.

166. **A.** Polypropylene is used frequently in vascular procedures.

167. **B.** Anaerobic means without oxygen.

168. **D.** To prevent foot drop, the peroneal nerve should be padded since it rests on the stirrups in the lithotomy position.

169. **B.** A primary characteristic of Graves' disease is hyperthyroidism. Other symptoms include weight loss, fatigue, palpitations, increased metabolic rate, and exophthalmos.

170. **C.** The Foley indwelling catheter drainage bag should be positioned lower than the level of the bladder.

171. **A.** The sutures of the skull are examples of synarthroses.

172. **D.** Laminar air flow is a high-flow unidirectional, air-blowing ventilation system.

173. **A.** Ketone bodies are produced through the catabolism of fats.

174. **D.** The principal reason for performing pre-operative skin prep is to remove transient flora and reduce resident flora.

175. **D.** The hypothalamus detects changes in temperature and triggers heat-conserving and generating activities, or activities that promote the loss of heat.

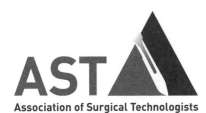
Directions: *Be sure to read each question carefully and select the best answer. You have four hours to complete the test. After finishing the test, review the answers and score your exam.*

In order to pass the CST examination, you must answer 118 questions correctly. If you achieved that score—congratulations! If not, take the time to identify what topics you struggled with and review the appropriate material.

1. **Which of the following clips is used for scalp hemostasis in cranial procedures?**

   o A. Raney

   o B. Filschie

   o C. Hemoclip

   o D. Backhaus

2. **The local freezing of diseased tissue to facilitate removal without bleeding is:**

   o A. Cryosurgery

   o B. Electrocautery

   o C. Diathermy

   o D. Harmonic scalpel

3. **In severe aortic stenosis, all of the following are indications of valve replacement except:**

   o A. Myocardial ischemia

   o B. Left ventricle hypertrophy

   o C. Palpitations

   o D. Angina

4. **In the event a child requires emergency surgery, but the parents cannot be located to sign the surgical consent:**

   o A. Consent is signed by a court of law

   o B. Consent is signed by two consulting physicians

   o C. No consent is required

   o D. Consent is signed by the surgeon

5. **Ethylene oxide sterilization destroys microbes by the process of:**

   o A. Alkylation

   o B. Osmosis

   o C. Oxidation

   o D. Cavitation

6. **What is the most common cause of aortic aneurysm?**

    o A. Thrombus
    o B. Embolus
    o C. Atherosclerosis
    o D. Hypotension

7. **What is used to determine the position of cannulated screws during repair of a femoral neck fracture?**

    o A. Broach
    o B. Guide pins
    o C. Canal reamer
    o D. Ruler

8. **The instruments shown below are used to dilate the:**

    o A. Urethra
    o B. Cervix
    o C. Coronary artery
    o D. Intranasal antrostomy

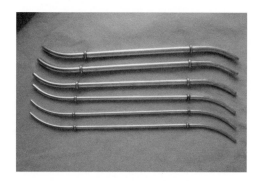

9. **Prior to being placed in the EtO sterilizer, items must:**

    o A. Not be heat sensitive
    o B. Be lubricated with oil
    o C. Have residual water on their surface
    o D. Be completely dry

10. **During general anesthesia induction, which sense is the last to be experienced by the patient?**

    o A. Touch
    o B. Taste
    o C. Hearing
    o D. Smell

11. **The purpose of creating an arteriovenous fistula is for:**

o A. Lavage

o B. Chemotherapy

o C. Hemodialysis

o D. Hemostasis

12. **What nerve is at greatest risk during a thyroidectomy?**

o A. Cervical sympathetic chain

o B. Inferior laryngeal

o C. Vagus

o D. Recurrent laryngeal

13. **Which nerve could be compressed against the humerus in the prone position?**

o A. Peroneal

o B. Tibial

o C. Brachial

o D. Radial

14. **What is the surgical procedure for reducing testosterone in prostate cancer?**

o A. Vasectomy

o B. Varicocelectomy

o C. Hydrocelectomy

o D. Orchiectomy

15. **What is the name of the retractor shown below?**

o A. Deaver

o B. Harrington

o C. Kelly

o D. Richardson

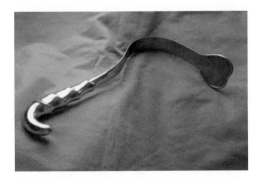

16. **If the broth in the steam sterilization biological indicator is yellow after incubation, what action should be taken?**

o A. Indicates autoclave chamber needs cleaning

o B. Items must be immediately recalled

o C. No action necessary

o D. Sterile items should be immediately used

17. **A specimen that is 5 centimeters is equal to:**

o A. 4 inches

o B. 2 inches

o C. 3 inches

o D. 5 inches

18. **Which of the following vessels arises from the right ventricle of the heart?**

o A. Descending aorta

o B. Ascending aorta

o C. Pulmonary vein

o D. Pulmonary artery

19. **The instrument below is used to:**

o A. Split muscle

o B. Resect tendon

o C. Extend incision

o D. Cut bone

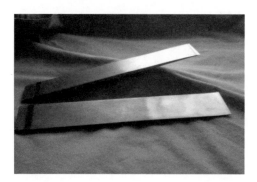

20. **Which area is prepped first when performing the skin prep for a skin grafting procedure?**

o A. Donor site

o B. Only recipient site

o C. Both sites together

o D. Recipient site

21. **Which of the following has legal significance in the mishandling of a bullet?**

   o   A.   Damage to tissue while removing specimen
   o   B.   Contaminating the specimen
   o   C.   Damaging ballistic markings
   o   D.   Tearing surgical gloves

22. **Which of the following procedures requires preoperative high-level disinfection of the endoscope?**

   o   A.   Bronchoscopy
   o   B.   Laparoscopy
   o   C.   Mediastinoscopy
   o   D.   Thoracoscopy

23. **Which of the following maintains the position of the uterus?**

   o   A.   Broad ligament
   o   B.   Suspensory ligament
   o   C.   Levator muscle
   o   D.   Pubic symphysis

24. **What device would the surgeon use to preserve facial motor and sensory functions during a parotidectomy?**

   o   A.   Ultrasound transducer
   o   B.   Mass spectrometer
   o   C.   Doppler probe
   o   D.   Nerve stimulator

25. **If the surgeon uses a knife blade to incise the oral mucosa, the preferred blade is:**

   o   A.   20
   o   B.   10
   o   C.   11
   o   D.   12

26. **The gravity steam sterilization process can be rendered ineffective if the:**

   o   A.   Air is removed
   o   B.   Steam quality is 97%
   o   C.   Temperature is below 250°
   o   D.   Packs are loosely arranged on cart

27. **A suture used to retract a structure to the side of the operative field is a/an:**

   o   A.   Retention suture
   o   B.   Traction suture
   o   C.   Bolster suture
   o   D.   Primary suture

28. **What must the circulating surgical technologist do when placing the patient in the supine position?**

    o A. Confirm ankles are not crossed
    o B. Place rolls under the axillae
    o C. Confirm chest is not compromised
    o D. Place a pillow between the knees

29. **What body system aids in the metastatic spread of cancer cells?**

    o A. Lymphatic
    o B. Reproductive
    o C. Respiratory
    o D. Limbic

30. **Which of the following is inserted into the tympanic membrane incision during a myringotomy?**

    o A. Fascial graft
    o B. PE tube
    o C. Weck-Cel® sponge
    o D. Speculum

31. **Which organelle contains digestive juices?**

    o A. Ribosome
    o B. Lysosome
    o C. Mitochondria
    o D. Nucleus

32. **During a thyroidectomy, if all parathyroid glands are accidentally removed, what complication will occur?**

    o A. Tetany
    o B. Bradycardia
    o C. Thyroid storm
    o D. Hemorrhage

33. **Which of the following surgical instruments is used to retract the lung?**

    o A. Glover
    o B. Kocher
    o C. Allison
    o D. Davidson

34. **Which of the following instruments would be used to remove nasal polyps?**

    o A. Antrum rasp
    o B. Krause nasal snare
    o C. Knight nasal scissors
    o D. Gruenwald nasal forceps

35. **What anatomical structure is Mersilene™ tape sutured around during a cerclage?**

o A. Ligaments
o B. Cervix
o C. Uterus
o D. Fallopian tubes

36. **What does the suffix -ectomy mean?**

o A. Incision
o B. Opening
o C. Anastomosis
o D. Excision

37. **What would the preoperative diagnosis be for an infant undergoing craniectomy?**

o A. Myelomeningocele
o B. Craniosynostosis
o C. Anencephaly
o D. Arteriovenous malformation

38. **Where is the anterior chamber of the eye located?**

o A. Posterior to the cornea and anterior to the iris
o B. Posterior to the cornea and anterior to the lens
o C. Posterior to the iris and anterior to the lens
o D. Posterior to the iris and anterior to the retina

39. **Which of the following would contraindicate preoperatively setting up the cell saver machine?**

o A. Patient received preoperative blood transfusion
o B. Patient is on preoperative steroids
o C. Sponges will be used during procedure
o D. Patient has cancer

40. **Which medication is contraindicated for patients with a history of malignant hyperthermia?**

o A. Succinylcholine
o B. Dantrolene
o C. Papaverine
o D. Vecuronium

41. **Which of the following is an incision into the tympanic membrane for the removal of accumulated fluid?**

o A. Otoplasty
o B. Tympanoplasty
o C. Stapedotomy
o D. Myringotomy

42. **Which of the following is not a requirement when a patient is placed in the prone position?**

- o A. Bolsters placed under axillae
- o B. Arms on armboards parallel to bed
- o C. Head placed on donut
- o D. Safety belt is placed below the knees

43. **A tissue specimen being sent to pathology for a frozen section is prepared by placing it into a:**

- o A. Basin of water
- o B. Jar with formalin
- o C. Jar with methylene blue
- o D. Container without preservative

44. **The body's first line of defense against infection is:**

- o A. Respiratory tract
- o B. Immune response
- o C. Intact skin
- o D. Hair follicles

45. **Which stapling device would be used to create an anastomosis during a low anterior resection?**

- o A. GIA
- o B. EEA
- o C. TA
- o D. LDS

46. **Packing material would be placed as a dressing after surgery on the:**

- o A. Rectum
- o B. Chest
- o C. Knee
- o D. Neck

47. **What is the lining of the thoracic cavity?**

- o A. Peritoneum
- o B. Pleura
- o C. Parietal
- o D. Pericardium

48. **What is the proper method for removing the knife blade from the handle when breaking down the Mayo stand?**

- o A. Throw handle with knife blade in sharps container
- o B. Use fingers
- o C. Do not remove and place handle in instrument tray
- o D. Use a heavy hemostat or needle holder

49. **What route of drug administration is parenteral?**

   o A. Intravenous
   o B. Sublingual
   o C. Rectal
   o D. Transdermal

50. **The vascular, fibrous covering of bone is the:**

   o A. Endosteum
   o B. Epiphysis
   o C. Aponeurosis
   o D. Periosteum

51. **What type of dressing would usually be used for a laparotomy procedure?**

   o A. Wet-to-wet
   o B. One-layer
   o C. Pressure
   o D. Bolster

52. **To prevent deep-vein thrombosis in the bariatric patient, what preoperative drug is given?**

   o A. Nitroglycerine
   o B. Heparin
   o C. Mannitol
   o D. Vitamin K

53. **Which space is entered during a thymectomy?**

   o A. Mediastinum
   o B. Interstitial
   o C. Pleural cavity
   o D. Retroperitoneum

54. **Femoral rasps are used for which of the following reasons:**

   o A. Expose the operative site
   o B. File the cortical bone
   o C. Prepare the intramedullary space for a prosthesis
   o D. Inject bone cement into the intramedullary space

55. **Which of the following is part of the immune system?**

   o A. Liver
   o B. Spleen
   o C. Pancreas
   o D. Thyroid

56. **What incision is frequently used for pediatric aortic coarctation repair?**

o A. Thoracoabdominal

o B. Median sternotomy

o C. Posterolateral thoracotomy

o D. Anterolateral thoracotomy

57. **Type and cross match for blood is completed:**

o A. On all hospital patients

o B. In the OR, just before the incision is made

o C. If blood loss with replacement is anticipated

o D. On all surgical patients

58. **The purpose of the kidney elevator is to:**

o A. Increase the intercostal spaces

o B. Stabilize the patient

o C. Facilitate respiration of the dependent lung

o D. Increase the space between the lower rib and iliac crest

59. **When storing information on the hard drive of a computer, what is clicked?**

o A. Open

o B. Delete

o C. Save

o D. Enter

60. **Which of the following is the proper method for handling disposable suction containers when turning over an OR?**

o A. Empty contents in hopper and place in waste container

o B. Place container in waste disposal

o C. Wipe down outside of container and place in biohazard bag for disposal

o D. Transport with instruments in case cart to decontamination room

61. **Which of the following can cause lumbosacral strain in the lithotomy position?**

o A. Stirrups not properly padded

o B. Arm boards placed beyond 90 degrees

o C. Safety strap is placed too tightly

o D. Buttocks extend past table break

62. **A midline xiphoid to pubis incision is commonly made for a/an:**

o A. Abdominal aortic aneurysmectomy

o B. Transverse colectomy

o C. Nephrectomy

o D. Appendectomy

63. **Which item listed below should the surgical technologist confirm is available for a nerve repair?**

   o A. CUSA
   o B. Nd:YAG Laser
   o C. Loupes
   o D. Cryotherapy unit

64. **How often should biological testing of EtO sterilization be conducted?**

   o A. Every load
   o B. Weekly
   o C. Monthly
   o D. Twice-a-week

65. **Which of the following is a liquid chemical sterilant often used for sterilizing endoscopes with a cycle time of 30 minutes?**

   o A. Isopropyl alcohol
   o B. Sodium hypochlorite
   o C. Peracetic acid
   o D. Glutaraldehyde

66. **When should the first closing sponge, sharp and instrument count be completed?**

   o A. Prior to closure of skin
   o B. Prior to closure of the body cavity
   o C. Prior to closure of the subcutaneous layer
   o D. Prior to closure of the muscle layer

67. **Which of the following skin preps is contraindicated for use around eyes and ears because of potential for corneal abrasions and ototoxicity?**

   o A. Parachlorometaxylenol
   o B. Chlorhexidine
   o C. Iodophors
   o D. Isopropyl alcohol

68. **A short-acting narcotic opioid given intramuscularly for preoperative sedation is:**

   o A. Meperidine
   o B. Midazolam
   o C. Morphine sulfate
   o D. Methylprednisolone

69. **The leg extensor muscles: rectus femoris, vastus lateralis, vastus medialis and the vastus intermedius are collectively called the:**

   o A. Popliteal fossa
   o B. Medial compartment
   o C. Quadriceps femoris
   o D. Peroneus longus

70. **Which of the following instruments is not a retractor used during a prostatectomy?**

o A. Denis-Browne

o B. Harrington

o C. Gil Vernet

o D. Mason-Judd

71. **What does the term -scopy mean?**

o A. Incision

o B. Viewing

o C. Probing

o D. Excision

72. **How many minutes should a Frazier suction tip be immediate-use sterilized (flash sterilized) in a gravity steam sterilizer?**

o A. 20

o B. 5

o C. 15

o D. 10

73. **Which of the following preoperative procedures should be completed for the diabetic patient?**

o A. Increase preoperative medications

o B. Increase preoperative insulin dose

o C. Preoperative meal to avoid hyperglycemia

o D. Antiembolic stockings placed on patient

74. **Induced hypothermia is typically associated with which of the following surgical specialties?**

o A. Orthopedic

o B. Gynecology

o C. Cardiothoracic

o D. Pediatric

75. **What block involves medication being injected into the subarachnoid space?**

o A. Regional

o B. Spinal

o C. Nerve

o D. Bier

76. **Which of the following conditions might require use of a Silastic® urethral catheter?**

o A. Prostatic hypertrophy

o B. Hypospadius

o C. Latex allergy

o D. Stress incontinence

77. **A patient receives preoperative instructions to remove nail polish to:**

o A. Allow completion of nuclear medicine study

o B. Prevent an infection

o C. Prevent pulse oximeter malfunction

o D. Allow arterial blood to be drawn

78. **How often should the steam sterilizing machine's strainer be cleaned?**

o A. Once-a-week

o B. During annual maintenance

o C. After each use

o D. Daily

79. **What is the smallest microorganism that requires a host cell for replication?**

o A. Amoeba

o B. Bacteria

o C. Fungi

o D. Virus

80. **Which surgeon might provide the operative exposure for the neurosurgeon in a transsphenoidal approach to the sella turcica?**

o A. Maxillofacial endodontist

o B. Otorhinolaryngologist

o C. Cardiothoracic surgeon

o D. Interventional radiologist

81. **An intraoperative mutagenic and carcinogenic hazard of laser use is:**

o A. Waste gases

o B. Laser plume

o C. Static electricity

o D. Infectious waste

82. **What type of solution is recommended for cleaning the OR floors during room turnover?**

o A. Isopropyl alcohol

o B. Detergent-disinfection

o C. Sodium hypochlorite

o D. Hydrogen peroxide

83. **Which of the following is used to remove resected prostatic tissue during a TURP?**

o A. Ellik

o B. Foley

o C. Pezzar

o D. Robinson

84. **A patient is instructed to be NPO for 8 hours prior to surgery to prevent:**

o A. Wound infection
o B. Ulcer
o C. Intestinal obstruction
o D. Aspiration

85. **The essential element of hemoglobin is:**

o A. Iron
o B. Sodium
o C. Nitrogen
o D. Oxygen

86. **In which procedure would the instrument shown below be used?**

o A. Lobectomy
o B. Laminectomy
o C. Nephrectomy
o D. Hysterectomy

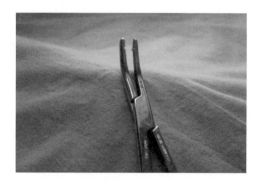

87. **A large, bony process found on the femur is a:**

o A. Trochanter
o B. Olecranon
o C. Condyle
o D. Tubercle

88. **Which of the following incisions would be performed for repair of a liver laceration?**

o A. Midline
o B. Pfannenstiel
o C. Transverse
o D. McBurney

89. **Just before the surgeon makes the skin incision, which of the following must be performed?**

o A. Time-out
o B. Postoperative orders are completed
o C. Mayo stand is correctly positioned
o D. Verify placement of EKG electrodes

90. **The pulse rate of pregnant patients:**

o A. Fluctuates

o B. Does not change

o C. Increases

o D. Decreases

91. **Which portion of the stomach is superior to the esophageal sphincter?**

o A. Antrum

o B. Pylorus

o C. Body

o D. Fundus

92. **A linen pack to be steam sterilized must not weigh more than:**

o A. 4 lbs

o B. 8 lbs

o C. 12 lbs

o D. 16 lbs

93. **The closing sponge count should be initiated at the:**

o A. Kick bucket

o B. Backtable

o C. Operative field

o D. Mayo stand

94. **During which of the following procedures is it imperative that the surgical technologist maintain the sterility of the backtable and Mayo stand until the patient is transported out of the OR?**

o A. Tonsillectomy

o B. Rhinoplasty

o C. Tympanoplasty

o D. Laminectomy

95. **Which of the following statements concerning peel-packs is correct?**

o A. Position peel packs plastic side facing plastic side

o B. When labeling with felt-tip marker write on the plastic side

o C. Use staples to close a peel pack

o D. Use chemical indicator tape to hold multiple items together

96. **Which two structures are identified and ligated during a cholecystectomy?**

o A. Hepatic duct and portal vein

o B. Cystic artery and cystic duct

o C. Right and left hepatic artery

o D. Splenic artery and splenic vein

97. **What is the primary responsibility of the first scrub surgical technologist during a cardiac arrest in the OR?**

o A. Assist the anesthesia provider

o B. Assist the circulator

o C. Protect the sterile field

o D. Give CPR to the patient

98. **What does pneumonectomy mean?**

o A. Incision into the bronchi

o B. Removal of the lung

o C. Incision into the trachea

o D. Removal of air from pleura

99. **How many hours must the steam biological indicator be incubated before recording the results?**

o A. 8

o B. 32

o C. 16

o D. 24

100. **Which of the following is responsible for causing transmission of spongiform encephalopathy?**

o A. Prion

o B. Fungi

o C. Bacteria

o D. Parasites

101. **The thyroid gland consists of right and left lobes joined by the:**

o A. Cricoid cartilage

o B. Isthmus

o C. Larynx

o D. Parathyroid gland

102. **A sustained contraction produced by rapid stimuli is called:**

o A. Tension

o B. Torsion

o C. Twitch

o D. Tetany

103. **What type of heart rate does tachycardia describe?**

o A. Absent

o B. Normal

o C. Fast

o D. Slow

104. **Which of the following would be the least likely complication of suprapubic prostatectomy?**

o   A.   Acute phlebitis

o   B.   Acute epididymitis

o   C.   Embolism

o   D.   Hemorrhage

105. **When is the surgical consent typically signed?**

o   A.   After preoperative medications are administered

o   B.   After the IV has been inserted

o   C.   Before preoperative medications are administered

o   D.   Just before general anesthesia is administered

106. **Which of the following is the order for postoperative case management?**

o   A.   Remove gown and gloves; don non-sterile gloves, remove drapes; break down backtable

o   B.   Remove gown; remove drapes; remove gloves; don non-sterile gloves; break down backtable

o   C.   Remove drapes; preserve sterile field until patient leaves OR; remove gown and gloves; don non-sterile gloves to break down backtable

o   D.   Remove drapes; remove gown and gloves; don non-sterile gloves; preserve sterile field until patient leaves OR; break down backtable

107. **What type of needle is used when suturing the skin?**

o   A.   Tapered

o   B.   Conventional cutting

o   C.   Side cutting

o   D.   Reverse cutting

108. **Which of the following ultrasonic devices can be used intraoperatively to assess the patency of arterial blood flow?**

o   A.   Lithotripter

o   B.   Stethoscope

o   C.   Spirometer

o   D.   Doppler probe

109. **The instrument shown below is used to:**

o A.   Cut bone
o B.   Smooth jagged ends of bone
o C.   Dissect tendon
o D.   Dissect periosteum from bone

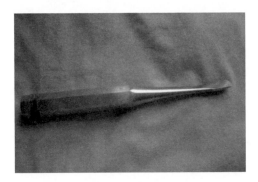

110. **The area of the brain that controls respiration is the:**

o A.   Corpus callosum
o B.   Medulla oblongata
o C.   Hypothalamus
o D.   Cerebellum

111. **Which of the following factors is used to determine the inflation pressure of a tourniquet?**

o A.   Previous surgeries
o B.   Length of surgery
o C.   Type of incision
o D.   Patient's age

112. **Which of the following describes the time from incision to the dressing application?**

o A.   Interoperative
o B.   Preoperative
o C.   Postoperative
o D.   Intraoperative

113. **At the end of a procedure, and after the patient has been transported out of the OR, the surgical technologist should remove the:**

o A.   Hair cover
o B.   Gloves
o C.   Mask
o D.   Gown

114. **The instrument shown below is used during a/an:**

o   A.   Gastrectomy

o   B.   Myringoplasty

o   C.   Thyroidectomy

o   D.   Rhinoplasty

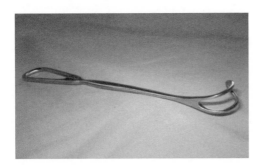

115. **What is considered the operative stage of anesthesia?**

o   A.   First

o   B.   Second

o   C.   Third

o   D.   Fourth

116. **When performing the surgical scrub, the hands and arms are considered:**

o   A.   Surgically clean

o   B.   Sterile

o   C.   Disinfected

o   D.   Sanitized

117. **Which of the following is an obstetric complication resulting from overstimulation of the clotting processes?**

o   A.   Disseminated intravascular coagulation

o   B.   Eclampsia

o   C.   Dystocia

o   D.   Placental abruption

118. **What does the term symbiosis mean?**

o   A.   Relationship between unlike species of organisms

o   B.   Organisms that destroy each other

o   C.   Aerobic organism

o   D.   Anaerobic organism

119. **Which of the following statements is true concerning cleaning OR walls between surgical procedures?**

  o A. Clean all walls floor to ceiling
  o B. Clean areas of wall splashed with blood or debris
  o C. Only clean walls splashed with blood or debris at end of day
  o D. Only clean walls at the end of the day

120. **Which anatomical structure is removed during a total hip arthroplasty?**

  o A. Trochanter
  o B. Femoral head
  o C. Fossa
  o D. Condyle

121. **What controls the arrow on your monitor?**

  o A. Mouse
  o B. Enter
  o C. Function keys
  o D. Shift

122. **Wound dressings should be opened:**

  o A. After last count is completed
  o B. During skin closure
  o C. After the skin incision is made
  o D. Just before skin closure is started

123. **A stent may be placed to identify the ureter during which of the following procedures?**

  o A. Endarterectomy
  o B. Hip arthroplasty
  o C. Right colectomy
  o D. Craniotomy

124. **A rapid-onset muscle relaxant used for intubation is:**

  o A. Morphine
  o B. Lanoxin®
  o C. Pitocin®
  o D. Anectine®

125. **A general consent form authorizes:**

  o A. Hazardous therapy
  o B. Receiving general anesthesia
  o C. Routine medical treatment
  o D. Experimental surgical treatment

126. **During which step of an abdominal hysterectomy would the instrument shown below be used?**

   o A. Enlarge peritoneal incision
   o B. Mobilize paracervical fascia
   o C. Dissect bladder from uterus
   o D. Make last cut to free the uterus

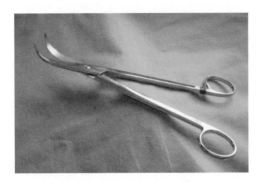

127. **Which of the following must be completed preoperatively if a patient underwent a barium study the day of surgery?**

   o A. Gastrostomy
   o B. Urinalysis
   o C. Enema
   o D. Colonoscopy

128. **Which of the following sutures is contraindicated in the presence of infection?**

   o A. Steel
   o B. Chromic
   o C. Silk
   o D. Polypropylene

129. **When the surgical technologist is breaking down the backtable, instruments with ratchets should be:**

   o A. Closed and placed in instrument tray for transport to decontamination
   o B. Placed in a basin with enzymatic solution in open position for transport to decontamination
   o C. Placed in a basin with saline for transport to decontamination
   o D. Run through the steam flash sterilizer before transport to decontamination

130. **The cup-like extensions of the renal pelvis that collect urine from the pyramids are:**

   o A. Papillae
   o B. Medulla
   o C. Cortex
   o D. Calyces

131. **Which of the following is a type of one-layer dressing?**

- o A. Steri-Strips™
- o B. Bulky
- o C. Pressure
- o D. Rigid

132. **Braided nonabsorbable sutures should not be used in infected wounds because suture crevices:**

- o A. Cause excessive postoperative pain
- o B. Can harbor bacteria that travel length of suture
- o C. Lead to pooling of tissue fluids
- o D. Cause necrosis of tissues

133. **What postoperative complication can result from excess or prolonged plantar flexion?**

- o A. Decubitus ulcer
- o B. Sciatica
- o C. Compartment syndrome
- o D. Foot drop

134. **What immediate postoperative complication most often occurs with pediatric patients?**

- o A. Airway difficulty
- o B. Electrolyte imbalance
- o C. Hypertension
- o D. Dysrhythmias

135. **Another name for a corneal transplant procedure is:**

- o A. Scleral buckle
- o B. Vitrectomy
- o C. Keratoplasty
- o D. Diathermy

136. **Fertilization normally occurs in the:**

- o A. Cervical os
- o B. Vaginal vault
- o C. Myometrium
- o D. Fallopian tube

137. **What is the name of the instrument shown below?**

o A. Dingman

o B. Kocher

o C. Pean

o D. Adson

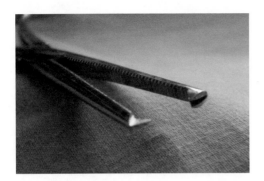

138. **The inner layer of an artery is the:**

o A. Viscera

o B. Adventitia

o C. Intima

o D. Media

139. **Which laser can be used on light and dark tissues?**

o A. Carbon dioxide

o B. Nd:YAG

o C. Excimer

o D. Argon

140. **What implant is used for individuals with sensorineural deafness?**

o A. Stapes implant

o B. Internal hearing aid

o C. Cochlear implant

o D. Fascial graft

141. **Splenectomy places the patient at an increased risk for:**

o A. Infection

o B. Cirrhosis

o C. Diabetes

o D. Jaundice

142. **In the presence of infection, the absorption rate of surgical gut is:**

o A. Increased

o B. Decreased

o C. Not affected

o D. Terminated

143. **Dark blood in the sterile field could indicate?**

o A. Tachycardia

o B. Hypovolemia

o C. Hypoxia

o D. Bradycardia

144. **Which instrument will the surgeon use to free the entrapped orbital fat during repair of an orbital floor fracture?**

o A. Chalazion

o B. Rongeur

o C. Freer

o D. Senn

145. **A urinary tract infection, following a cystoscopy, is an example of what type of infection?**

o A. Recurrent

o B. Healthcare-associated infection

o C. Latent

o D. Community-acquired infection

146. **Which of the following is a type of meniscal tear?**

o A. Greenstick

o B. Bucket handle

o C. Capsular

o D. Comminuted

147. **Which surgical procedure may require a suprapubic catheter to drain the urinary bladder?**

o A. Appendectomy

o B. Cloward procedure

o C. Prostatectomy

o D. Caesarean section

148. **Which one of these microorganisms is least likely to be associated with wound infections?**

o A. *Escherichia coli*

o B. *Staphylococcus*

o C. *Clostridium perfringens*

o D. *Treponema pallidum*

149. **Liquid agents used to reduce microorganisms on the patient's skin are:**

o A. Germicidals

o B. Sporicidals

o C. Disinfectants

o D. Antiseptics

150. **Which closed wound drainage device requires being connected to a bulb evacuator?**

o A. Stryker

o B. Jackson-Pratt

o C. Hemovac

o D. Cigarette drain

151. **What term refers to items remaining sterile indefinitely until the wrapping is compromised?**

o A. Time-related sterility

o B. Contaminated-related sterility

o C. Shelf-life sterility

o D. Event-related sterility

152. **Which of the following veins would be harvested during a CABG?**

o A. Femoral

o B. Popliteal

o C. Subclavian

o D. Saphenous

153. **When incubated, the EtO biological indicator can be read after:**

o A. 48 hours

o B. 72 hours

o C. 12 hours

o D. 24 hours

154. **The structure that facilitates the exchange of nutrients and wastes between the fetus and mother is the:**

o A. Endometrium

o B. Umbilical cord

o C. Placenta

o D. Amniotic fluid

155. **When helping to turn over an OR between patients, the surgical technologist should:**

o A. Clean around the furniture

o B. Use a clean mop head

o C. Clean overhead lights after last procedure of day

o D. Wipe down entire walls

156. **Vitrectomy is the removal of the:**

o A. Opaque lenses

o B. Trabecular meshwork

o C. Iris

o D. Gel from the eye

157. **When using EtO sterilization, the recommended aeration time for an aerator set at 140°F is:**

o A. 8 hours

o B. 10 hours

o C. 12 hours

o D. 24 hours

158. **Where should the biological indicator test be placed on the steam sterilizer cart?**

o A. Middle second shelf

o B. Bottom front

o C. Top front

o D. Top back

159. **Which of the following vessels empties into the right atrium?**

o A. Pulmonary vein

o B. Aortic arch

o C. Superior vena cava

o D. Pulmonary artery

160. **Knife blades should be loaded onto the handle with:**

o A. Needle holder

o B. Allis clamp

o C. DeBakey forceps

o D. Sterile gloved hands

161. **Which of the following vitamins is essential for the clotting process?**

o A. D

o B. B

o C. K

o D. A

162. **From where do most intracranial aneurysms arise?**

o A. Ventricular system

o B. Cavernous sinus

o C. Internal carotid

o D. Circle of Willis

163. **Which of the following types of equipment would require preoperative draping by the surgical technologist?**

o A. Video monitor

o B. ESU

o C. Arthroscope

o D. C-arm

164. **What dietary substance enhances the production of collagen?**

   o A. Carbohydrates
   o B. Fats
   o C. Protein
   o D. Vitamins

165. **The normal range of intraoperative pressure for the insufflator during a laparoscopy is:**

   o A. 3–6 mm Hg
   o B. 6–9 mm Hg
   o C. 9–12 mm Hg
   o D. 12–15 mm Hg

166. **Where should the EtO biological indicator be placed in the load?**

   o A. Side
   o B. Front
   o C. Back
   o D. Center

167. **What is the proper way to remove a patient from the lithotomy position?**

   o A. Lower legs together slowly in unison
   o B. Lower stirrups, then remove legs
   o C. Lower legs together quickly in unison
   o D. Lower each leg separately

168. **What procedure should the first scrub surgical technologist set up for when a female patient is undergoing a repair for a cystocele and rectocele?**

   o A. Abdominal hysterectomy
   o B. Anterior and posterior colporrhaphy
   o C. D & C
   o D. Myomectomy

169. **Which vein drains the small intestine?**

   o A. Gastric
   o B. Inferior vena cava
   o C. Hepatic portal
   o D. Hepatic

170. **What specialized retractors are used during a rotator cuff repair?**

   o A. Hibbs
   o B. Bankart
   o C. Hohmann
   o D. Taylor

171. **The concave notch of the kidney through which the ureter exits is the:**

   o A. Calyx
   o B. Pyramid
   o C. Hilum
   o D. Capsule

172. **The large artery found posterior to the knee is the:**

   o A. Tibial
   o B. Popliteal
   o C. Geniculate
   o D. Femoral

173. **Proper placement of the Foley catheter is confirmed prior to balloon inflation by which of the following?**

   o A. Removal of 5 mL of air from balloon
   o B. Collapse of catheter lumen
   o C. Secure connection to drainage bag
   o D. Urine flowing out of catheter

174. **Which portion of the small intestine joins to the large intestine?**

   o A. Jejunum
   o B. Duodenum
   o C. Ileum
   o D. Cecum

175. **Which tank would be brought into the OR if a surgical technologist is preparing an oscillating saw?**

   o A. Nitrous oxide
   o B. Compressed nitrogen
   o C. Freon
   o D. Compressed air

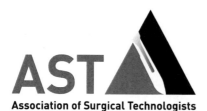

ASSOCIATION OF SURGICAL TECHNOLOGISTS
PRACTICE EXAM #5 ANSWER KEY

1.	A	31.	B	61.	D	91.	D	121.	A	151.	D
2.	A	32.	A	62.	A	92.	C	122.	A	152.	D
3.	C	33.	C	63.	C	93.	C	123.	C	153.	D
4.	B	34.	B	64.	A	94.	A	124.	D	154.	C
5.	A	35.	B	65.	C	95.	B	125.	C	155.	B
6.	C	36.	D	66.	B	96.	B	126.	D	156.	D
7.	B	37.	B	67.	B	97.	C	127.	C	157.	A
8.	B	38.	A	68.	A	98.	B	128.	C	158.	B
9.	D	39.	D	69.	C	99.	D	129.	B	159.	C
10.	C	40.	A	70.	B	100.	A	130.	C	160.	A
11.	C	41.	D	71.	B	101.	B	131.	A	161.	C
12.	D	42.	D	72.	D	102.	D	132.	B	162.	D
13.	D	43.	D	73.	D	103.	C	133.	D	163.	D
14.	D	44.	C	74.	C	104.	A	134.	A	164.	C
15.	B	45.	B	75.	B	105.	C	135.	C	165.	D
16.	B	46.	A	76.	C	106.	C	136.	D	166.	D
17.	B	47.	B	77.	C	107.	D	137.	B	167.	A
18.	D	48.	D	78.	D	108.	D	138.	C	168.	B
19.	D	49.	A	79.	D	109.	D	139.	A	169.	C
20.	A	50.	D	80.	B	110.	B	140.	C	170.	B
21.	C	51.	C	81.	B	111.	D	141.	A	171.	C
22.	A	52.	B	82.	B	112.	D	142.	A	172.	B
23.	A	53.	A	83.	A	113.	D	143.	C	173.	D
24.	D	54.	C	84.	D	114.	C	144.	C	174.	C
25.	D	55.	B	85.	A	115.	C	145.	B	175.	B
26.	C	56.	C	86.	D	116.	A	146.	B		
27.	B	57.	C	87.	A	117.	A	147.	C		
28.	A	58.	D	88.	A	118.	A	148.	D		
29.	A	59.	C	89.	A	119.	B	149.	D		
30.	B	60.	C	90.	C	120.	B	150.	B		

1. **A.** Bleeding from the scalp can be profuse. The Raney scalp system is used to control the hemorrhage during craniotomy procedures.

2. **A.** A cryotherapy unit uses liquid nitrogen, Freon, or carbon dioxide gas to provide extreme cold through a probe directed at the diseased tissue to destroy it without harming adjacent tissue.

3. **C.** Aortic stenosis blocks the complete flow of blood from the left ventricle into the aorta, causing left ventricle hypertrophy, hypertension, myocardial ischemia, angina and eventually heart failure.

4. **B.** When the parent(s) or legal guardian(s) cannot be located or contacted, the surgeon will inform two physicians who must agree the patient needs surgery and sign the surgical consent.

5. **A.** EtO is an alkylating agent that destroys microbes by interfering with normal metabolism of protein and reproduction.

6. **C.** Atherosclerosis is the most common cause of aortic aneurysm.

7. **B.** Three guide pins are placed in the femoral head and cannulated screws placed over each pin.

8. **B.** The Heaney or Hegar uterine dilators are used to dilate the cervix during a D & C procedure.

9. **D.** Items to be placed in the EtO sterilizer must be completely clean, dry and free from lubricating oils; EtO gas cannot penetrate the lubricants.

10. **C.** The last sense to be suppressed during general anesthesia is hearing.

11. **C.** Arteriovenous fistula is the direct connection of an artery and vein to create vascular access for long-term hemodialysis.

12. **D.** The recurrent laryngeal nerve must be identified and protected from injury during a thyroidectomy. Injury to the nerve can result in temporary or permanent hoarseness or loss of voice.

13. **D.** The radial nerve innervates the muscles on the back of the arm. If the forearm hangs over the side of the bed, it could be compressed against the humerus.

14. **D.** To decrease the testosterone level in the presence of prostate cancer, an orchiectomy procedure is performed.

15. **B.** The Harrington "Heart" retractor is a large retractor with smooth edges making it ideal to retract abdominal organs.

16. **B.** Yellow broth indicates the microbes weren't killed during the sterilization cycle, and the items from the load are not sterile. The items must be immediately recalled and reprocessed.

17. **B.** 2.54 centimeters is equal to 1 inch; therefore, 5 centimeters is about 2 inches (1.97 to be exact).

18. **D.** The pulmonary artery arises from the right ventricle.

19. **D.** The Lambotte osteotome is available in varying widths and has a sharp end making it ideal for cutting bone.

20. **A.** The donor site is prepped first and is "clean;" the recipient site is prepped last and is considered "dirty" if it is an open wound or potentially contains cancer cells.

21. **C.** Bullets must be carefully handled. Do not use forceps or clamps because it could damage the ballistic markings.

22. **A.** Because the endoscope is inserted through the mouth into the bronchial tubes, a bronchoscopy is considered a clean procedure.

23. **A.** The broad, uterosacral, cardinal and round ligaments maintain the position of the uterus.

24. **D.** The nerve stimulator produces small electric currents that are applied to tissue and aid in identifying essential nerves.

25. **D.** One option for the cold dissection of the tonsils is the use of the #12 knife blade.

26. **C.** The temperature must reach 250° F when using a gravity displacement sterilizer.

27. **B.** Traction sutures are used to retract a structure that cannot be retracted with a handheld or self-retaining retractor.

28. **A.** When a patient is placed in the supine position, the ankles and legs should not be crossed to avoid impairment of circulation and damage to the peroneal nerve.

29. **A.** Lymphatic system aids in the metastatic spread of cancer cells.

30. **B.** Ventilation or pressure equalizing (PE) tube is inserted into the incision to facilitate pressure equalization.

31. **B.** Lysosomes contain the enzyme lysozyme that destroys foreign substances ingested by the cell.

32. **A.** Tetany is characterized by severe cramps, convulsions and twitching of the muscles, and extreme flexion of the joints caused by a low level of calcium.

33. **C.** The Allison lung retractor is a non-traumatic retractor that is used specifically for the lung.

34. **B.** The Krause nasal snare is loaded with a flexible wire that is placed around the nasal polyp. The snare is tightened around the polyp to dissect free.

35. **B.** Cervical cerclage, also called Shirodkar's procedure, involves placing a large diameter Dacron® or Mersilene™ tap around the cervix at the level of the internal os.

36. **D.** The suffix -ectomy means excision.

37. **B.** Craniosynostosis is a condition when infant suture lines prematurely close.

38. **A.** The anterior chamber is a cavity of the eyeball that lies behind the cornea and in front of the iris.

39. **D.** If cancer is suspected or known, the cell saver machine will not be used since it cannot wash or remove cancers cells from the blood.

40. **A.** Certain agents may trigger malignant hyperthermia including succinylcholine.

41. **D.** Myring/o is a combining form meaning tympanic membrane. Myringotomy is an incision into the tympanic membrane.

42. **D.** When placing a patient in the prone position a safety belt placed below the knees is not a requirement.

43. **D.** The tissue designated for a frozen section must be kept dry; solutions such as formalin, water or saline will alter the freezing process.

44. **C.** The body's first line of defense against infection is skin that has no cuts, scrapes, etc.

45. **B.** The EEA is a type of intraluminal stapler that is used during resection and reanastomosis of the distal colon or rectum.

46. **A.** Packing material is used to provide hemostasis, support the wound and eliminate dead space. It is used for rectal, nasal and vaginal procedures.

47. **B.** The pleural membrane lines the thoracic cavity.

48. **D.** The knife blade should never be removed using the fingers. A heavy hemostat, such as a Kelly, or needle holder, should be used to remove the blade and thrown into the sharps container.

49. **A.** Parenteral refers to the methods when drugs are administered with a needle.

50. **D.** The fibrous covering that covers bone and provides some degree of protection is the periosteum.

51. **C.** Normally, a pressure dressing is applied for a laparotomy procedure to provide wound support, eliminate dead space and reduce edema.

52. **B.** Heparin is usually administered subcutaneously 30 minutes before the procedure begins to aid in preventing DVT.

53. **A.** The thymus is located in the mediastinum between the sternum and aorta.

54. **C.** The femoral rasps are graduated in size from small to large; the surgeon uses a back-and-forth motion to remove cancellous bone and enlarge the canal.

55. **B.** Lymph nodes, tonsils and spleen are all part of the immune system and help the body fight infection.

56. **C.** The approach for a pediatric aortic coarctation repair is made through the left posterolateral thoracotomy into the third or fourth intercostal space.

57. **C.** If blood loss for a particular procedure is anticipated, the patient's blood will be preoperatively typed-and-cross matched.

58. **D.** Turning the patient from the supine to kidney position, the patient is positioned so that the lower iliac crest is just below the lumbar break. The kidney elevator is raised to increase the space between the lower rib and iliac crest.

59. **C.** Frequently saving a document is important so the information is not lost in case the computer malfunctions or there is a power outage.

60. **C.** The outside of the disposable suction container should be wiped down and placed in a bag with the biohazard symbol for disposal.

61. **D.** Buttocks extending past the table break can cause lumbosacral strain in the lithotomy position.

62. **A.** The incision for an AAA is xiphoid to pubis in order to gain as much exposure of the artery as possible, including bifurcation.

63. **C.** Loupes are a type of magnifying lenses worn by a surgeon during delicate procedures such as plastic surgery and neurosurgery;

64. **A.** It is recommended a BI be included with every EtO sterilization load.

65. **C.** Peracetic acid is a strong sterilant that is used with the Steris machine and has a total cycle time of approximately 30 minutes.

66. **B.** As soon as the peritoneum or other type of body cavity (ie, uterus) starts to be closed, the surgical technologist should initiate the first closing count with the circulator. The count should be completed prior to the cavity being completely closed.

67. **B.** Chlorhexidine is contraindicated using for facial preparation.

68. **A.** Meperidine (Demerol®) is a short-acting opioid narcotic given intramuscularly for premedication.

69. **C.** The quadriceps femoris, largest muscle in the body, consists of four separate muscles: rectus femoris, vastus lateralis, vastus medialis, and vastus intermedius.

70. **B.** A Harrington retractor would not be used during a prostatectomy due to its large size.

71. **B.** "-scopy" (o/scopy) is the suffix that means viewing.

72. **D.** Since the Frazier suction tip has a lumen, a residual of distilled water should be left inside the lumen and immediate-use sterilized (flash sterilized) for 10 minutes.

73. **D.** Diabetic patients often have poor circulation of the lower extremities and are prone to thromboembolism. Antiembolic stockings are worn by the patient.

74. **C.** Induced hypothermia is the deliberate lowering of the body's core temperature and is an adjunctive therapy for use during open-heart surgery.

75. **B.** Intrathecal (spinal) block is a method of anesthesia when medication is injected into the subarachnoid space affecting a portion of the spinal cord.

76. **C.** If a patient has latex allergies, a Silastic urethral catheter may be required.

77. **C.** Nail polish changes the color of the pulse oximeter light beam causing malfunction.

78. **D.** The strainer is located at the bottom front of the autoclave chamber and should be cleaned daily.

79. **D.** Viruses are a non-living particle that completely rely on the host cell for survival.

80. **B.** Otorhinolaryngologists are commonly called ear, nose and throat surgeons, and might assist by providing the operative exposure for the neurosurgeon in a transphenoidal approach to the sella turcica.

81. **B.** When using a laser, surgical plume is produced that has been shown through research to contain mutagenic and carcinogenic particles. The surgical team should wear the proper PPE.

82. **B.** An EPA-registered detergent-disinfection solution is recommended for use in cleaning the OR floor during turnover in preparation for the next procedure.

83. **A.** The Ellik evacuator is used intermittently by the surgeon to remove resected prostatic tissue during a TURP. A Toomey syringe can be used for the same purpose.

84. **D.** The presence of food or fluids in the stomach predisposes the patient to vomiting due to all the drugs and anesthesia which can cause pneumonia and death.

85. **A.** Iron is an essential ingredient of hemoglobin, the oxygen-carrying protein in blood.

86. **D.** Heaney hysterectomy and Heaney-Ballantine hysterectomy clamps, collectively referred to as ligament clamps, are heavy, tissue clamps that are excellent for placing across the uterine ligaments during dissection.

87. **A.** A trochanter is a large, bony process found on the femur.

88. **A.** The initial incision is a long midline incision that may be extended to a thoracoabdominal incision.

89. **A.** Before the surgeon is handed the knife handle to make the skin incision, the operative team should conduct a "time-out" to confirm correct patient, correct surgery site and correct procedure.

90. **C.** The pulse rate of pregnant patients increases to compensate for the increase in circulatory volume that is necessary to support the fetus.

91. **D.** The fundus is the portion of the stomach located above the level of the upper esophageal sphincter.

92. **C.** A linen pack that is assembled within the healthcare facility must not weigh more than 12 pounds.

93. **C.** The recommended sequence for performing the closing count is operative field, Mayo stand, backtable, basin, off the sterile field.

94. **A.** Procedures that involve the oral cavity and neck predispose the patient to complications such as hemorrhage and airway difficulties, and an emergency tracheostomy may have to be performed.

95. **B.** When using a felt-tip marker to label the peel pack, write only on the plastic side; ink can leak through the paper causing the items to be unsterile.

96. **B.** The cystic artery and then cystic duct are double clamped, double ligated and divided.

97. **C.** The surgical technologist's primary role during a cardiac arrest in the OR is to protect the sterile field; however, he/she may be called upon to provide chest compressions or provide artificial respiration.

98. **B.** Removal of the lung is a pneumonectomy.

99. **D.** The steam BI must be incubated for 24 hours before the reading can be recorded.

100. **A.** A prion is a protein substance that is responsible for causing transmissible spongiform encephalopathy.

101. **B.** The two lobes of the thyroid gland are joined by the isthmus that lies just above the second tracheal ring.

102. **D.** Tetany is a sustained contraction of a muscle produced by several rapid stimuli.

103. **C.** Tachycardia refers to a rapid heart and/or pulse rate.

104. **A.** Hemorrhage, embolism and acute epididymitis are all postoperative complications of a suprapubic prostatectomy.

105. **C.** The surgical consent must be signed prior to the patient receiving any medications/drugs that could alter the patient's mental status, causing the inability to fully understand the surgeon's explanations and what he/she is signing.

106. **C.** The optimal sequence is remove items from drapes and remove drapes; move Mayo stand and back table away from OR table and preserve sterility until patient leaves OR; remove the gown and gloves; don non-sterile exam gloves and break down the backtable and Mayo stand.

107. **D.** Reverse cutting needles are used for closing the skin, because the needle has a flat edge in the direction of pull which decreases the damage to the skin.

108. **D.** The Doppler is an ultrasonic device used to assess the flow of blood through arteries and veins. A sterile probe can be used within the sterile field.

109. **D.** The name Key periosteal elevator provides how the instrument is used. During open procedures, the Key is used to dissect or "elevate" the periosteum from the bone.

110. **B.** The medulla oblongata is responsible for controlling respirations.

111. **D.** The three factors used to determine the inflation pressure of a tourniquet are patient's age, circumference of the extremity and systolic blood pressure.

112. **D.** The intraoperative phase occurs during the time the surgical procedure is being performed, starting with the skin incision and ending with the placement of the sterile dressings.

113. **D.** After the drapes are removed and patient transported out of the OR, the surgical technologist removes the gown and then gloves.

114. **C.** The Green retractor is often used during thyroidectomy and other procedures when gentle retraction of friable tissue is needed.

115. **C.** The operative stage of general anesthesia is the third stage.

116. **A.** The surgical scrub is performed to remove as many microbes as possible and render the hands and arms surgically clean.

117. **A.** Pregnancy can trigger disseminated intravascular coagulation (DIC), a pathology when the normal clotting mechanisms fail.

118. **A.** Symbiosis is a constant relationship between two or more unlike species of organisms.

119. **B.** During room turnover, spot clean the wall(s) that were splashed with blood or debris.

120. **B.** The femoral head and neck are resected and replaced by the femoral component.

121. **A.** The mouse is used to move the cursor to different areas on the screen or within a document.

122. **A.** The circulator should not open and dispense the sterile dressings until the final closing count is completed and verified as being correct.

123. **C.** One of the complications of any type of colon resection (ie, left hemicolectomy, transverse hemicolectomy, abdominoperineal resection) includes ureteral injury. To help prevent the injury, a ureteral stent may be inserted to identify the ureter.

124. **D.** Succinylcholine chloride (Anectine®) is a rapid-onset muscle relaxant used for intubation in short cases.

125. **C.** The general consent is for treatment defined in the broadest terms including general medical treatment and diagnostic procedures.

126. **D.** The last three steps of the procedure entail cutting the uterosacral ligaments, cut the uterus with the knife in preparation for removal, and final cut with the Jorgenson scissors to remove the uterus.

127. **C.** A preoperative enema must be performed to eliminate the barium, because it predisposes the patient to postoperative fecal impaction.

128. **C.** Silk sutures are not used in the presence of infection.

129. **B.** Instruments should be placed in a basin and covered with sterile water, enzymatic or detergent solution and unratcheted for transport to the decontamination room.

130. **D.** The cup-like extensions of the kidney pelvis that collect urine are calyces.

131. **A.** Steri-Strips™ are a type of one-layer dressing used to maintain approximation of the wound edges. They may be used alone or as part of another dressing.

132. **B.** Multiple-strand or braided suture has the characteristic called capillarity, which is conducive to harboring bacteria that can travel the length of the suture. Consequently, multiple-strand suture should not be used in the presence of infection.

133. **D.** A patient placed in the supine position must be protected from foot drop. If the feet extend beyond the end of the OR table, they must be supported to prevent a stretch injury.

134. **A.** Airway complications are the most common concern when a pediatric patient is emerging from anesthesia and during the postoperative period.

135. **C.** Kerat/o is a combining form meaning cornea. Keratoplasty refers to a corneal transplant.

136. **D.** Fertilization of an ovum usually takes place in the fallopian tubes.

137. **B.** The Kocher clamp is easily distinguished by the single tooth on the end, making it a good instrument for grasping heavy tissue.

138. **C.** The inner layer of an artery is called the intima or tunica intima.

139. **A.** Carbon dioxide energy is absorbed by the cellular water content. The absorption does not depend on tissue color or consistency.

140. **C.** A cochlear implant is a prosthetic replacement of the cochlea located in the inner ear. It is implanted in individuals suffering from sensorineural deafness.

141. **A.** The spleen functions as part of the immune system, and its removal can impair the immunologic response.

142. **A.** The absorption rate of plain surgical gut and chromic gut increases when an infection is present.

143. **C.** Hypoxia is a deficiency in oxygen and is indicated by dark blood.

144. **C.** The periorbital fat and other entrapped tissue are released with the use of the Freer elevator or scissors and tissue forceps.

145. **B.** Healthcare-acquired infections (HAI) are associated with urinary tract infections following cystoscopy.

146. **B.** The meniscus can sustain various types of tears, but a common type is the bucket handle characterized by an incomplete longitudinal tear.

147. **C.** A suprapubic catheter is placed into the bladder through an opening in the abdominal wall and may be required after a prostatectomy.

148. **D.** *Treponema pallidum* is associated with syphilis.

149. **D.** Antiseptics are solutions used by surgical team members to perform the surgical scrub as well as used on the patient for skin preparation.

150. **B.** The Jackson-Pratt is a type of active drain that consists of a drainage tube and an evacuator, shaped like a bulb, often called the grenade.

151. **D.** Event-related sterility means that the sterility of an item is determined by how it is handled and that contamination is event related, not time related.

152. **D.** The two vessels commonly harvested for use during a CABG are the internal mammary artery and saphenous vein.

153. **D.** The EtO BI can be read after 24 hours. However, it must be incubated for 48 hours.

154. **C.** The placenta provides an exchange of nutrients and wastes between the fetus and mother and secretes the hormones necessary to maintain the pregnancy.

155. **B.** A new mop-head should be used each time an OR is being turned-over for the next procedure.

156. **D.** Vitrectomy is a microsurgical procedure when the vitreous gel is removed. It is the initial step to repair retinal disorders.

157. **A.** The recommended aeration at 140° F is for a minimum of 8 hours.

158. **B.** The BI test should be placed at the bottom front of the sterilizer cart since that is the coldest point of the autoclave chamber.

159. **C.** The right atrium receives blood from three veins: coronary sinus, superior vena cava, inferior vena cava.

160. **A.** The surgical technologist should practice sharps safety and always load the knife blade onto the handle, typically using a needle holder.

161. **C.** Vitamin K is essential for the clotting process.

162. **D.** The most common site of cerebral aneurysm arise in the Circle of Willis.

163. **D.** The upper portion of the C-arm is positioned over the sterile drapes covering the patient. The surgical technologist should cover the upper arm with a specialized sterile C-arm drape.

164. **C.** Collagen fibers consist of the protein collagen which has the highest percentage in the body.

165. **D.** The normal intraoperative range of pressure for laparoscopy is 12–15 mm Hg.

166. **D.** The EtO BI should be placed in the center of the load on its side since that is the location most difficult for the gas to reach.

167. **A.** When moving a patient out of the lithotomy position, the legs must be lowered together slowly to the OR table to avoid injury to the muscles and nerves of the lumbar region of the back and prevent hypotension.

168. **B.** Cystoceles and rectoceles are prolapses of the bladder and rectum into the vaginal vault. The anterior repair is for the cystocele and posterior repair for the rectocele.

169. **C.** The hepatic portal vein drains blood from the pancreas, spleen, stomach, intestines and gallbladder.

170. **B.** The Bankart shoulder retractors were specifically developed for use during shoulder procedures.

171. **C.** The hilum, also called the renal hilum, is a notch near the center of the concave border of the kidney through which the ureter leaves.

172. **B.** The popliteal artery is located behind the knee joint.

173. **D.** Urine flowing out of a Foley catheter confirms proper placement prior to balloon inflation.

174. **C.** The ileum is the portion of the small intestine that joins the large intestine.

175. **B.** Most large power instruments, such as saws and drills, use either electricity (rechargeable power batteries) or nitrogen.

AST

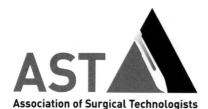
This bonus basic science review section is intended to measure your knowledge of basic anatomy and physiology, microbiology, pharmacology and medical terminology. The national certification examination includes 50 basic science questions which could be challenging, because you probably studied this information early in your program. Use this section to refresh your knowledge of this important area.

Read each question carefully and be sure you understand the question. After completing each bonus test, score your exam and review the questions you answered accurately and those you did not.

Utilize this bonus review section to identify the areas you need to focus on and study where needed.

1. **What is the name of the condition when the foreskin of the penis cannot be retracted to normal position?**

   o A. Epispadias
   o B. Hydrocele
   o C. Cryptorchidism
   o D. Phimosis

2. **What shape are bacilli?**

   o A. Rod-shaped
   o B. Round
   o C. Curved
   o D. Spiral

3. **What type of stapling device is used to perform low anterior anastomosis?**

   o A. EEA
   o B. GIA
   o C. TA
   o D. LDS

4. **Which division of the autonomic nervous system is responsible for the "fight or flight" response?**

   o A. Visceral
   o B. Sympathetic
   o C. Parasympathetic
   o D. Somatic

5. **Surgical puncture of the joint space with a needle for synovial fluid drainage is called:**

- o A. Arthroscopy
- o B. Arthroplasty
- o C. Arthrography
- o D. Arthrocentesis

6. **Excessive secretion of growth hormones in adults causes:**

- o A. Hepatomegaly
- o B. Pituitary dwarfism
- o C. Splenomegaly
- o D. Acromegaly

7. **Oophorectomy is the surgical removal of the:**

- o A. Fallopian tube
- o B. Corpus luteum
- o C. Uterus
- o D. Ovary

8. **Which term refers to voluntary skeletal muscle?**

- o A. Striated
- o B. Cardiac
- o C. Visceral
- o D. Smooth

9. **The suffix "-pexy" means:**

- o A. Rule, order
- o B. Fixation, to put in place
- o C. Eat, swallow
- o D. Attraction for

10. **Which part of the neuron conducts impulses away from the cell body?**

- o A. Axon
- o B. Dendrite
- o C. Soma
- o D. Ganglion

11. **The prefix "pseudo-" means:**

- o A. False
- o B. Again
- o C. Under
- o D. With

12. **Disruption of previously sutured tissue layers is:**

   o A. Dehiscence

   o B. Sinus tract

   o C. Prolapse

   o D. Fistula

13. **An inanimate object upon which pathogens may be conveyed is referred to as a:**

   o A. Bioburden

   o B. Fomite

   o C. Flora

   o D. Vector

14. **The hormone responsible for the development and maintenance of the female secondary sex characteristics is:**

   o A. Progesterone

   o B. Inhibin

   o C. Prolactin

   o D. Estrogen

15. **Which of the following muscles is not a component of the rotator cuff of the shoulder?**

   o A. Infraspinatus

   o B. Subscapularis

   o C. Trapezius

   o D. Supraspinatus

16. **A foreign substance that stimulates the production of antibodies is a/an:**

   o A. Antigen

   o B. Androgen

   o C. Endotoxin

   o D. Exotoxin

17. **The suffix "-lysis" means:**

   o A. Tumor, mass

   o B. Softening

   o C. Breakdown, destruction

   o D. Enlargement

18. **Diatrizoate megulmine (Hypaque® or Renografin®) or lothalamute meglumine (Conray®) are examples of:**

   o A. Staining agents

   o B. Diuretics

   o C. Dyes

   o D. Contrast media

19. **The small intestine is divided into how many sections?**

   o A. 2
   o B. 3
   o C. 4
   o D. 5

20. **Epidural anesthesia involves the administration of an anesthetic agent into the space surrounding the:**

   o A. Spinal cord
   o B. Pia mater
   o C. Dura mater
   o D. Subarachnoid space

21. **The electrical component of the heart that causes contraction of the ventricles is the:**

   o A. SA node
   o B. Purkinje fibers
   o C. AV node
   o D. Bundle of His

22. **Which of the following is an action of antimicrobials?**

   o A. Inhibit the microbial immune system
   o B. Inhibit bacterial cell wall synthesis
   o C. Promote cell metabolism
   o D. Promote protein synthesis

23. **The anatomical landmark located at the proximal, lateral portion of the femoral shaft is the:**

   o A. Lateral epicondyle
   o B. Medial condyle
   o C. Lesser trochanter
   o D. Greater trochanter

24. **The primary stablizing ligament of the knee which is attached to the posterior lateral:**

   o A. Medial collateral
   o B. Posterior cruciate
   o C. Anterior cruciate
   o D. Lateral collateral

25. **What type of bone are carpal bones?**

   o A. Short
   o B. Flat
   o C. Sesamoid
   o D. Irregular

26. **The prefix "para-" means:**

o A. Surrounding

o B. Through

o C. Near, beside

o D. Many, much

27. **A direct or indirect inguinal hernia indicates a tear in:**

o A. Transversalis fascia

o B. Cooper's ligament

o C. Scarpa's fascia

o D. Fascia lata

28. **The bending of the foot downward at the ankle joint is called:**

o A. Eversion

o B. Plantar flexion

o C. Inversion

o D. Dorsiflexion

29. **Which of the following vertebrae have ribs attached?**

o A. Cervical

o B. Lumbar

o C. Sacral

o D. Thoracic

30. **Which organ produces bile?**

o A. Small intestine

o B. Gallbladder

o C. Liver

o D. Pancreas

31. **Which of the following describes spherically shaped bacteria?**

o A. L-form

o B. Cocci

o C. Prion

o D. Bacilli

32. **Lack of control over urination is called:**

o A. Micturition

o B. Retention

o C. Incontinence

o D. Urinary meatus

33. **Which agent is used to perform an intraoperative cholangiogram?**

   o A. Hypaque meglumine (Hypaque®)
   o B. Acetic acid
   o C. Indigo carmine
   o D. Methylene blue

34. **What does the thymus gland produce for the immune response?**

   o A. Antigens
   o B. T-cells
   o C. Lymphocytes
   o D. Interferon

35. **Which cranial nerve arises from the medulla and innervates the cervical, thoracic and abdominal regions?**

   o A. IX
   o B. X
   o C. XI
   o D. XII

36. **The total number of vertebrae in the adult is:**

   o A. 26
   o B. 29
   o C. 33
   o D. 37

37. **The medical term for the chest is:**

   o A. Diaphragm
   o B. Pleura
   o C. Thorax
   o D. Mediastinum

38. **Cholecystectomy is removal of the:**

   o A. Urinary bladder
   o B. Stomach
   o C. Gallbladder
   o D. Colon

39. **Which of the following are the cells of the bone?**

   o A. Osteocytes
   o B. Osteoblastoma
   o C. Osteoclasts
   o D. Osteoblasts

40. **Which of the following is the medical term for the calf muscle?**

o A. Plantaris

o B. Gastrocnemius

o C. Sartorius

o D. Quadriceps

41. **The suffix -malacia refers to:**

o A. Enlargement

o B. Seizures

o C. Hardening

o D. Softening

42. **For which tissue type would a cutting needle be contraindicated?**

o A. Intestine

o B. Eye

o C. Tendon

o D. Skin

43. **Which of the following would affect normal wound healing?**

o A. Peripheral vascular disease

o B. Skin prep

o C. Penicillin allergy

o D. Clean wound

44. **The nuclear material of the bacterial cell has been found to:**

o A. Be a combination of ATP and RNA

o B. Exist as two or more chromosomes

o C. Exist as a single molecule of DNA

o D. Have a distinct nuclear membrane

45. *Escherichia coli* **is normally present inside which of the following anatomical structures?**

o A. Posterior pharynx

o B. Stomach

o C. Colon

o D. Lower esophagus

46. **Which of the following nerves innervates the breast?**

o A. Pudendal

o B. Brachial plexus

o C. Axillary

o D. Anterior thorax

47. **In which fossa is the cerebellum located?**

o A. Medial

o B. Lateral

o C. Posterior

o D. Anterior

48. **Omnipaque, a water soluble iodine-based contrast medium is used for:**

o A. Schiller's test

o B. Angiography

o C. Isotope scanning

o D. Chromotubation

49. **Tetanus and botulism are caused by organisms of the genus:**

o A. Vibrio

o B. Clostridium

o C. Bacillus

o D. Streptococcus

50. **Which of the following is a phase of first intention wound healing?**

o A. Contraction

o B. Granulation

o C. Maturation

o D. Chronic

51. **Which of the following sutures is a polyester fiber suture?**

o A. Dexon™

o B. Vicryl™

o C. Nurolon™

o D. Ethibond®

52. **Growth in a long bone occurs at the:**

o A. Epiphyseal plate

o B. Perpendicular plate

o C. Femoral canal

o D. Medullary canal

53. **Air in the pleural cavity is:**

o A. Pneumothorax

o B. Pleurisy

o C. Atelectasis

o D. Hemothorax

54. **The initial result of fertilization of gametes is a/an:**

   o A. Fetus
   o B. Zygote
   o C. Blastocyst
   o D. Embryo

55. **The thorax is formed posteriorly by the:**

   o A. Sternum
   o B. Twelve pair of ribs
   o C. Diaphragm
   o D. Twelve thoracic vertebrae

56. **The seventh cranial nerve is called the:**

   o A. Trigeminal
   o B. Facial
   o C. Glossopharyngeal
   o D. Optic

57. **What does the term cephalalgia mean?**

   o A. Pelvic pain
   o B. Intestinal pain
   o C. Backache
   o D. Headache

58. **The prefix "brady-" means:**

   o A. Two
   o B. Slow
   o C. Down
   o D. Against

59. **Which of the following is a parenteral route of drug administration?**

   o A. Topical
   o B. Rectal
   o C. Oral
   o D. Intravenous

60. **Misalignment or deviation of the eye is:**

   o A. Strabismus
   o B. Cataracts
   o C. Entropion
   o D. Astigmatism

61. **Following administration, most of the drugs are converted to less active or inactive substances called:**

   o A. Urea
   o B. Ions
   o C. Metabolites
   o D. Compounds

62. **Hemorrhaging that occurs between the skull and outer meningeal covering is a/an:**

   o A. Epidural hematoma
   o B. Intracerebral hematoma
   o C. Subdural hematoma
   o D. Subarachnoid hematoma

63. **If a suture strand hangs or extends over the sterile table edge, the surgical technologist in the scrub role should:**

   o A. Watch it closely so that no one comes near it
   o B. Use it anyway as long as nothing unsterile touched it
   o C. Consider the suture contaminated and discard it
   o D. Pull it back onto the table to prevent it from becoming contaminated

64. **The term pharmacodynamics means:**

   o A. Excretion of drugs
   o B. Interaction between drugs and target cells
   o C. Absorption and distribution of drugs
   o D. Metabolism of drugs

65. **A relationship between two kinds of organisms that live together for mutual benefit is called:**

   o A. Parasitism
   o B. Commensalism
   o C. Phagocytosis
   o D. Mutualism

66. **Hemostasis means to:**

   o A. Arrest blood flow
   o B. Create blood flow
   o C. Bypass an occluded blood vessel
   o D. Maintain within normal limits

67. **What type of tissue is cartilage?**

   o A. Epthelial
   o B. Connective
   o C. Nervous
   o D. Muscle

68. **Heparin is classified as a/an:**

- o A. Coagulant
- o B. Anticoagulant
- o C. Antibiotic
- o D. Muscle relaxant

69. **Enlargement of the veins of the spermatic cord is a:**

- o A. Hydrocele
- o B. Rectocele
- o C. Cystocele
- o D. Varicocele

70. **Red blood cells are also known as:**

- o A. Leukocytes
- o B. Erythrocytes
- o C. Lymphocytes
- o D. Thrombocytes

71. **The standard volume for an Asepto syringe is approximately:**

- o A. 60 cc
- o B. 90 cc
- o C. 120 cc
- o D. 200 cc

72. **In which of the following processes does destruction of spores occur?**

- o A. Sterilization
- o B. Gestation
- o C. Disinfection
- o D. Decontamination

73. **Which of the following systemic conditions affects the ophthalmic system?**

- o A. Arthritis
- o B. Lymphoma
- o C. Diabetes
- o D. Cirrhosis

74. **The pectoral girdle is formed by the:**

- o A. Scapula and glenoid
- o B. Coxal bones
- o C. Clavicle and humerus
- o D. Scapula and clavicle

75. **Tubercle bacillus is found in the:**

- o A. Cerebrospinal fluid
- o B. Intestinal tract
- o C. Respiratory tract
- o D. Synovial fluid

76. **Which of the following bones does not articulate with another bone?**

- o A. Hyoid
- o B. Ulna
- o C. Temporal
- o D. Parietal

77. **The adrenal cortex secretes:**

- o A. Urine
- o B. Insulin
- o C. Epinephrine
- o D. Hormones

78. **Rickettsial diseases of humans are transmitted by:**

- o A. Infected human contact
- o B. Contaminated food consumption
- o C. Rodent contact
- o D. Tick bite

79. **Antibiotics are commonly administered intraoperatively by which of the following routes?**

- o A. Orally
- o B. Rectally
- o C. Intravenous
- o D. Intramuscular

80. **The scroll-like ridges on the lateral walls of the nasal cavity are called the:**

- o A. Hard palate
- o B. Palantine tonsils
- o C. Nasal conchae
- o D. Tympanic membrane

81. **What drug is added to a local anesthetic to decrease bleeding?**

- o A. Epinephrine
- o B. Cocaine
- o C. Thrombin
- o D. Hyaluronidase

82. **Inherited deficiencies of coagulation in which bleeding occurs spontaneously after minor trauma is called:**

   o A. Pernicious anemia

   o B. Tay-Sachs disease

   o C. Erythroblastosis fetalis

   o D. Hemophilia

83. **When an anesthetized patient's position is changed from Trendelenberg to dorsal recumbent, he/she should be moved slowly to prevent:**

   o A. Circulatory depression

   o B. Hypothermia

   o C. Hypertension

   o D. Muscle strain

84. **The cranial nerve that innervates the larynx and pharynx is the:**

   o A. Glossopharyngeal

   o B. Hypoglossal

   o C. Vagus

   o D. Accessory

85. **Cefazolin (Ancef®) is a/an:**

   o A. Diuretic

   o B. Steroid

   o C. Mydriatic

   o D. Antibiotic

86. **All of the following are inhalation agents except:**

   o A. Ethrane

   o B. Nitrous oxide

   o C. Fluothane

   o D. Atropine

87. **Bolsters are used with retention sutures to:**

   o A. Facilitate easy removal

   o B. Prevent unequal tension

   o C. Facilitate visualization

   o D. Prevent skin lacerations

88. **Pulse oximetry involves the noninvasive measurement of which of the following arterial blood saturation levels?**

   o A. Carbon dioxide

   o B. Oxygen

   o C. Nitrous oxide

   o D. Propofol

89. Which bone of the skull is most superior?

o A. Frontal

o B. Occipital

o C. Parietal

o D. Temporal

90. A dissociative drug that produces a short-term, trance-like state and hallucinations is:

o A. Sodium pentathol

o B. Ketamine (Ketalar®)

o C. Succinylcholine (Anectine®)

o D. Fentanyl (Sublimaze®)

91. Which of the following is a commonly used type of anesthesia for obstetric and perineal procedures?

o A. Epidural

o B. Topical

o C. Cryoanesthesia

o D. Bier Block

92. The basic unit of length in the metric system is the:

o A. Millimeter

o B. Centimeter

o C. Meter

o D. Micrometer

93. The process by which leukocytes engulf and destroy bacteria is called:

o A. Pinocytosis

o B. Commensalism

o C. Parasitism

o D. Phagocytosis

94. The motor-sensory cranial nerve that innervates the tongue is the:

o A. Hypoglossal

o B. Facial

o C. Vestibulocochlear

o D. Olfactory

95. Which of the following is a type of degenerative joint disease?

o A. Osteoarthritis

o B. Osteoporosis

o C. Osteomalacia

o D. Osteosarcoma

96. **The accumulation of cerebrospinal fluid in the brain of children is known as:**

o A. Huntington's chorea

o B. Meningocele

o C. Spina bifida

o D. Hydrocephalus

97. **A thick-walled, highly resistant body formed within a bacterial cell is a/an:**

o A. Cyst

o B. Nucleus

o C. Capsule

o D. Spore

98. **The C-shaped rings of the trachea are composed of:**

o A. Ligament

o B. Bone

o C. Cartilage

o D. Tendon

99. **An enzyme extracted from bovine blood that is used as a topical hemostatic agent is:**

o A. Collagen

o B. Tannic acid

o C. Oxytocin

o D. Thrombin

100. **The 126 bones that compose the upper and lower extremities of the body is called the:**

o A. Vertebral column

o B. Appendicular skeleton

o C. Pelvic girdle

o D. Axial skeleton

101. **The absorption of a drug depends upon all of the following, except:**

o A. Dosage of the drug

o B. Route of administration of the drug

o C. Time of the day when the drug is given

o D. Type of drug preparation

102. **An angulated fracture of the distal radius is a/an:**

o A. Greenstick

o B. Spiral

o C. Colles'

o D. Potts

103. **Which cranial nerve is responsible for the sense of smell?**

   o A. I
   o B. II
   o C. III
   o D. IV

104. **What is the purpose of the surgical hand scrub?**

   o A. Negate the need for wearing gown and gloves
   o B. Remove bioburden from contaminated skin
   o C. Reduce the microbial count
   o D. Sterilize the hands and arms

105. **The end of a long bone is the:**

   o A. Diaphysis
   o B. Periosteum
   o C. Epiphysis
   o D. Endosteum

106. **A combining form meaning kidney is:**

   o A. Ur/o
   o B. Cyst/o
   o C. Rhin/o
   o D. Ren/o

107. **The tail-like distal fibers of the spinal cord form the:**

   o A. Cauda equina
   o B. Conus medullaris
   o C. Lumbar plexus
   o D. Filum terminale

108. **What is an external mechanical method of hemostasis?**

   o A. Pneumatic tourniquet
   o B. Ultrasonic scalpel
   o C. Cotton pledgets
   o D. Hemostatic clamp

109. **A dilation of the arterial wall is called:**

   o A. Atherosclerosis
   o B. Aneurysm
   o C. Fistula
   o D. Embolism

110. **Organisms that are highly resistant to destruction and can survive a harsh environment are:**

o A. Cocci

o B. Spores

o C. Aerobes

o D. Anaerobes

111. **The suffix "-rrhea" means:**

o A. Birth, labor

o B. Breathing

o C. Flow, discharge

o D. To pour

112. **Where are the malleus, incus, and stapes located?**

o A. Mastoid sinus

o B. Tympanic membrane

o C. Bony labyrinth

o D. Middle ear

113. **A miotic drug is:**

o A. Pilocarpine

o B. Scopolamine

o C. Homatropine

o D. Atropine

114. **Neurons that conduct impulses to the spinal cord and brain are called:**

o A. Peripheral

o B. Efferent

o C. Afferent

o D. Unipolar

115. **A microscopic blood exam that estimates the percentages of each type of white cell within a sample is called:**

o A. Plasma cell count

o B. Platelet count

o C. Differential blood count

o D. Erthyrocyte count

116. **Which of the following natural sutures is treated with a salt solution to decrease the rate of absorption?**

o A. Plain gut

o B. Surgical silk

o C. Chromic gut

o D. Stainless steel

117. **When the vertebral column develops an abnormal lateral curve, the condition is called:**

- o A. Lordosis
- o B. Scoliosis
- o C. Spondylosis
- o D. Kyphosis

118. **Which statement concerning sterile technique is false?**

- o A. Only the surface level of a table with a sterile cover is considered sterile
- o B. Flaps on peel-packs must be pulled apart, never torn
- o C. The last flap of a sterile package wrapped envelope style should be opened toward the unsterile person
- o D. An opened sterile bottle of saline or water may be recapped carefully

119. **Multiplication of a cell into two separate cells is known as:**

- o A. Binary fission
- o B. Fusion
- o C. Pleomorphism
- o D. Separatism

120. **The rounded portion of the uterus superior to the uterine tubes is called the:**

- o A. Fundus
- o B. Isthmus
- o C. Cervix
- o D. Body

121. **Which of the following medications inhibits blood coagulation?**

- o A. Calcium
- o B. Warfarin
- o C. Vitamin K
- o D. Neosynephrine

122. **A drug used to reverse the effect of muscle relaxants is:**

- o A. Narcan
- o B. Fentanyl
- o C. Morphine
- o D. Prostigmin®

123. **The major difference between procaryotic cells and eucaryotic cells is:**

- o A. Procaryotic cells have a well-defined nuclear membrane whereas eucaryotic cells do not
- o B. Eucaryotic cells have a well-defined nuclear membrane whereas procaryotic cells have no true nucleus
- o C. Eucaryotic cells are usually found in pathogenic bacteria
- o D. There is very little difference between eucaryotic and procaryotic cells

124. **The inner lining of the heart is called the:**

o A. Myocardium

o B. Endocardium

o C. Pericardium

o D. Epicardium

125. **Which of the following conditions exists if a patient has a white blood cell count of 12,500?**

o A. Edema

o B. Hemophilia

o C. Infection

o D. Leukopenia

126. **What is the function of hemoglobin?**

o A. Regulate temperature

o B. Fight infection

o C. Initiate clotting

o D. Carry oxygen

127. **Which of the following is an electrical recording of heart activity?**

o A. Electrocardiogram

o B. Electroencephalogram

o C. Ventriculogram

o D. Myelogram

128. **The primary mode of airborne bacteria in the operating room is the:**

o A. Surgical team

o B. Patient

o C. Endotracheal tube

o D. Instruments

129. **Which of the following is a salivary gland?**

o A. Pituitary

o B. Pineal

o C. Parotid

o D. Pancreas

130. **Which virus is the precursor to Acquired Immunodeficiency Syndrome?**

o A. HBV

o B. HIV

o C. HPV

o D. HAV

131. **Which of the following is not an action of stapling devices?**

   o   A.   Anastomose

   o   B.   Transect

   o   C.   Ligate

   o   D.   Retract

132. **The acromion process is part of which bone?**

   o   A.   Clavicle

   o   B.   Scapula

   o   C.   Humerus

   o   D.   Ulna

133. **What term means the rupture of a wound with protrusion of abdominal contents?**

   o   A.   Dehiscence

   o   B.   Evisceration

   o   C.   Disruption

   o   D.   Herniation

134. **The thick, crescent-shaped pads of cartilage that rest on the upper articular surface of the tibia are the:**

   o   A.   Capsules

   o   B.   Bursae

   o   C.   Menisci

   o   D.   Condyles

135. **Which portion of the sterile gown is considered non-sterile once it has been donned?**

   o   A.   Arms up to 2 inches above the elbows

   o   B.   Table level to 2 inches below the neck line

   o   C.   Axillary region

   o   D.   Side tie

136. **How many millimeters does one meter equal?**

   o   A.   25

   o   B.   50

   o   C.   100

   o   D.   1,000

137. **The heel bone of the foot is called the:**

   o   A.   Tarsal

   o   B.   Phalanges

   o   C.   Calcaneus

   o   D.   Metatarsal

138. **The shaft of a bone is known as the:**

   o   A.   Metaphysis
   o   B.   Condyle
   o   C.   Diaphysis
   o   D.   Endosteum

139. **A virus that infects a bacterial cell is called a/an:**

   o   A.   Viroid
   o   B.   Chromatid
   o   C.   Bacteriophage
   o   D.   Inclusion

140. **Another name for spongy bone is:**

   o   A.   Callus
   o   B.   Cancellous
   o   C.   Cortical
   o   D.   Compact

141. **Which suture size would be used for ophthalmic procedures?**

   o   A.   8-0
   o   B.   2-0
   o   C.   0
   o   D.   2

142. **The true ribs articulate anteriorly with the:**

   o   A.   Pectoral girdle
   o   B.   Scapula
   o   C.   Thoracic vertebrae
   o   D.   Sternum

143. **The suffix "-trophy" means:**

   o   A.   Wasting
   o   B.   Lack of strength
   o   C.   Development, nourishment
   o   D.   Fibrous connective tissue

144. **Which intention of healing occurs in a wound with a large loss of tissue?**

   o   A.   First
   o   B.   Second
   o   C.   Third
   o   D.   Fourth

145. **Which class of surgical wound has the highest rate of infection?**

  o   A.   I
  o   B.   II
  o   C.   III
  o   D.   IV

146. **Atrophy means:**

  o   A.   Death of tissue
  o   B.   Increase in muscle fiber size
  o   C.   Without
  o   D.   Wasting away

147. **Which of the following types of anaerobic bacteria is the cause of gas gangrene?**

  o   A.   *Fusobacterium*
  o   B.   *Clostridium perfringens*
  o   C.   *Clostridium botulinum*
  o   D.   *Bacteroides fragillis*

148. **What is the pharmacological classification of Furosemide?**

  o   A.   Diuretic
  o   B.   Adrenergic
  o   C.   Hormone
  o   D.   Hemostatic

149. **Which of the following has the highest tensile strength but poor handling qualities?**

  o   A.   Silk
  o   B.   Polyester fiber
  o   C.   Dacron®
  o   D.   Stainless steel

150. **Lasix® is a/an:**

  o   A.   Antibiotic
  o   B.   Steroid
  o   C.   Coagulant
  o   D.   Diuretic

151. **The ability of a microbe to move by itself can be provided by:**

  o   A.   Cilia
  o   B.   L-form
  o   C.   Capsule
  o   D.   Exotoxin

152. **The most common side effects of drugs include all of the following except:**

o A. Diarrhea and constipation

o B. Hemorrhage and edema

o C. Dizziness and drowsiness

o D. Nausea and vomiting

153. **The arousal from general anesthesia after cessation of the anesthetic agent is called:**

o A. Induction

o B. Enticement

o C. Emergence

o D. Excitement

154. **What is another name for a stick tie?**

o A. Suture reel

o B. Free needle

o C. Suture ligature

o D. Free tie

155. **Childbirth labor may be induced by:**

o A. Lidocaine (Xylocaine)

o B. Diazoxide (Hyperstat IV)

o C. Ergonovine (Ergotrate®)

o D. Oxytocin (Pitocin®)

156. **The finger-like projections on the end of the fallopian tubes are:**

o A. Phalanges

o B. Cilia

o C. Metacarpals

o D. Fimbriae

157. **Which of the following is a "basic right" for correct drug handling?**

o A. Drug and dosage

o B. Manufacturer

o C. Type of syringe

o D. Who mixed the drug

158. **Which of the following is a seminal tract accessory gland that surrounds the urethra?**

o A. Ejaculatory ducts

o B. Testes

o C. Prostate

o D. Adrenal

159. **Agar is a/an:**

  o A. Disease-causing microbe

  o B. Microscope used for studying bacteria

  o C. Plastic dish used for growing microorganisms

  o D. Agent used to solidify growth media in the microbiology laboratory

160. **What is the trade name for polyglactin 910?**

  o A. Ethibond®

  o B. Vicryl™

  o C. PDS®

  o D. Dexon™

161. **The prefix that means above or upon is:**

  o A. Ad-

  o B. Dia-

  o C. Epi-

  o D. Trans-

162. **A tendon is defined as a structure that attaches:**

  o A. Bone to bone

  o B. Muscle to muscle

  o C. Muscle to bone

  o D. Nerve to bone

163. **The upper portion of the stomach is called the:**

  o A. Rugae

  o B. Antrum

  o C. Body

  o D. Fundus

164. **Which type of needle point would be selected for use on tendon or skin?**

  o A. Spatula

  o B. Blunt

  o C. Cutting

  o D. Taper

165. **The left coronary artery divides into the:**

  o A. Posterior interventricular and marginal

  o B. Middle and marginal

  o C. Anterior interventricular and circumflex

  o D. Middle and great cardiac

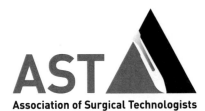

ASSOCIATION OF SURGICAL TECHNOLOGISTS

BONUS SCIENCE REVIEW QUESTIONS #1

1	D	31	B	61	C	91	A	121	B	151	A
2	A	32	C	62	A	92	C	122	D	152	B
3	A	33	A	63	C	93	D	123	B	153	C
4	B	34	B	64	B	94	A	124	B	154	C
5	D	35	B	65	D	95	A	125	C	155	D
6	D	36	A	66	A	96	D	126	D	156	D
7	D	37	C	67	B	97	D	127	A	157	A
8	A	38	C	68	B	98	C	128	A	158	C
9	B	39	A	69	D	99	D	129	C	159	D
10	A	40	B	70	B	100	B	130	B	160	B
11	A	41	D	71	C	101	C	131	D	161	C
12	A	42	A	72	A	102	C	132	B	162	C
13	B	43	A	73	C	103	A	133	B	163	D
14	D	44	C	74	D	104	C	134	C	164	C
15	C	45	C	75	C	105	C	135	C	165	C
16	A	46	D	76	A	106	D	136	D		
17	C	47	C	77	D	107	A	137	C		
18	D	48	B	78	D	108	A	138	C		
19	B	49	B	79	C	109	B	139	C		
20	C	50	C	80	C	110	B	140	B		
21	B	51	D	81	A	111	C	141	A		
22	B	52	A	82	D	112	D	142	D		
23	D	53	A	83	A	113	A	143	C		
24	C	54	B	84	C	114	C	144	B		
25	A	55	D	85	D	115	C	145	D		
26	A	56	B	86	D	116	C	146	D		
27	A	57	D	87	D	117	B	147	B		
28	B	58	B	88	B	118	D	148	A		
29	D	59	D	89	C	119	A	149	D		
30	C	60	A	90	B	120	A	150	D		

1. **D.** Phimosis is a pathology in which the prepuce cannot be retracted over the glans penis.

2. **A.** Bacilli are recognized by their rod-shape.

3. **A.** EEA is a stapling device used to perform lower anterior anastomosis.

4. **B.** The sympathetic nervous system is a division of the ANS that causes a physiological response to danger or emergencies.

5. **D.** Arthrocentesis involves placing a needle into the joint to withdraw synovial fluid for diagnostic purposes or remove excess fluid.

6. **D.** Overactive GH-producing cells cause acromegaly characterized by widening of the bones of the face, hands and feet.

7. **D.** Oophorectomy is the removal of one or both ovaries.

8. **A.** Skeletal muscle tissue is striated; skeletal muscle is voluntary.

9. **B.** The suffix pexy means to fixate such as orchiopexy.

10. **A.** An axon is the cytoplasmic process of a neuron that conducts impulses away from the cell body.

11. **A.** Pseudo- means false, such as pseudoaneurysm.

12. **A.** Dehiscence is the partial or total separation of layers of tissue.

13. **B.** Fomites are inanimate objects, such as the backtable and Mayo stand, that harbor microbes.

14. **D.** Estrogen is responsible for the development and maintenance of the female secondary sex characteristics.

15. **C.** Surrounding the shoulder joint is the rotator cuff that consists of four muscles: infraspinatus, teres minor, subscapularis and supraspinatus.

16. **A.** An antigen is a foreign substance in the body that initiates the immune response with the production of antibodies.

17. **C.** Lysis means separation, destruction or loosening; it can be used a a suffix or stand alone word.

18. **D.** Hypaque®, Renografin® and Conray® are types of contrast media used for the visualization of vessels and organs during X-ray examinations.

19. **B.** The small intestine is divided into the duodenum, jejunum (middle section), and ileum (distal section).

20. **C.** Epidural anesthesia involves administering an anesthetic agent into the tissues located right above the dura mater.

21. **B.** The electrical impulses from the bundle of His enter the Purkinje fibers and the fibers focus the impulses to the apex of the left ventricle resulting in contraction.

22. **B.** The action of the majority of antibiotics is inhibiting cell wall synthesis during multiplication.

23. **D.** The greater trochanter is located on the upper, lateral part of the upper shaft of the femur; it serves as the insertion for the gluteus medius and minimus.

24. **C.** The ACL is attached to the posterior lateral condyle of the femur and midline notch (intercondylar) of the tibia.

25. **A.** Carpal bones are a type of short bone that aid in the movement of the wrist.

26. **A.** Para- means surrounding such as in paranasal sinuses, the cavities that surround the nasal cavity.

27. **A.** The transversalis fascia is the primary focus of inguinal hernias; a hernia occurs when the fascia ruptures or tears and is repaired during surgery.

28. **B.** Plantar flexion is bending the foot downward at the ankle joint.

29. **D.** There are 12 thoracic vertebrae and the 12 ribs that articulate with each thoracic vertebra.

30. **C.** The liver is a complex organ that carries out multiple physiological activities, including producing bile.

31. **B.** Coccus (sing.form; cocci, pl.) refers to round-shaped bacteria.

32. **C.** Incontinence is the involuntary lack of control of urination; one type is stress incontinence.

33. **A.** Hypaque is a type of contrast agent used to outline biliary structures during surgery.

34. **B.** The thymus gland functions in immunity by producing T-cells.

35. **B.** The vagus (X) is the cranial nerve that emerges from the medulla, passes through the skull, and descends through the neck region into the thorax and abdominal region.

36. **A.** During early development the number of vertebrae is 33; when the sacral and coccygeal regions fuse the adult vertebrae numbers 26.

37. **C.** The thorax refers to the chest or thoracic cavity.

38. **C.** Cholecystectomy is removal of the gallbladder primarily as a laparoscopic procedure.

39. **A.** Bone cells are called osteocytes.

40. **B.** The gastrocnemius is the superficial muscle of the calf.

41. **D.** The suffix -malacia means softening such as osteomalacia.

42. **A.** A cutting needle would not be used on friable intestinal tissue.

43. **A.** Chronic or acute diseases, such as PVD, negatively affect the ability of a wound to heal.

44. **C.** The bacterial cell contains a single strand of DNA that is unique to each bacterial species.

45. **C.** *E. coli* colonizes within the colon and obtains nutrients from the food humans eat, and produce vitamin K.

46. **D.** The nerves of the breast are cutaneous nerves from the anterior thorax.

47. **C.** The cerebellum is positioned in the inferior and posterior area of the cranial cavity.

48. **B.** Omnipaque is a contrast dye that is injected into the artery or vein during an angiography.

49. **B.** Tetanus and botulism are caused by Gram-positive anaerobic bacteria.

50. **C.** Three phases of first intention wound healing are: lag (inflammatory response), proliferation and maturation (differentiation phase).

51. **D.** Ethibond Excel® is an example of a polyester fiber suture.

52. **A.** The epiphyseal plate is the area of a bone where growth occurs until early adulthood.

53. **A.** Pneumothorax is the entry of air into the pleural cavity due to blunt or penetrating trauma; it displaces the lung which can collapse due to inability to expand.

54. **B.** The result of fertilization of gametes is a zygote.

55. **D.** The twelve pair of ribs articulate posteriorly with twelve thoracic vertebrae.

56. **B.** The seventh cranial nerve is the facial nerve that transmits impulses to the pons.

57. **D.** Cephalalgia is another term for headache.

58. **B.** Brady- means slow such as bradycardia.

59. **D.** Parenteral means by injection; it includes intradermal, subcutaneous, intramuscular and intravenous.

60. **A.** Strabismus is the misalignment or deviation of the eye(s) that includes crossed eyes and wall eyes.

61. **C.** Biotransformation of drugs usually occurs in the liver, breaking down products of metabolism into metabolites.

62. **A.** The bleeding from an epidural hematoma rips the dura away from the skull resulting in more hemorrhaging.

63. **C.** Any item that extends or falls below the table edge is considered non-sterile.

64. **B.** Pharmacodynamics is the study of the interaction of drugs with the target cells of living organisms.

65. **D.** Mutualism is when both microbes benefit from one another.

66. **A.** Hemostasis is stopping hemorrhage by pressure, ligation, or with hemostatic agents.

67. **B.** Connective tissue is the most abundant tissue in the body; examples include cartilage, bone, ligaments and blood.

68. **B.** Heparin sodium prevents clot formation; it is used during vascular procedures.

69. **D.** Varicocele is due to varicosities of the veins that drain the testes and the scrotum swells.

70. **B.** The medical term for RBCs is erythrocytes that contain hemoglobin.

71. **C.** The Asepto syringe is the most frequently used irrigator that holds about 120cc.

72. **A.** Sterilization is the destruction of spores and microorganisms on inanimate objects.

73. **C.** Diabetes mellitus places an individual at a higher risk for developing retinopathy that results in blindness.

74. **D.** The two pectoral girdles, also called shoulder girdles, consist of the clavicle and scapula.

75. **C.** Tuberculosis is caused by *Mycobacterium tuberculosis* and usually infects the lungs.

76. **A.** The hyoid bone is a part of the axial skeleton and is the only bone in the body that does not articulate with another bone; it supports the tongue and aids in keeping the larynx continuously open.

77. **D.** The adrenal cortex secretes steroid type of hormones that are important in the control of fluid and electrolyte balance.

78. **D.** Rickettsia are gram-negative, pleomorphic coccobacilli transmitted to humans by bites of infected ticks or mites, or feces of infected lice or fleas.

79. **C.** Antibiotics are often administered intravenously by the anesthesia provider.

80. **C.** The two chambers of the nasal cavity have a series of bony projections called the nasal conchae or turbinates.

81. **A.** Epinephrine is a vasoconstrictor that is often mixed with local anesthetics to provide hemostasis and to keep the local from being rapidly absorbed.

82. **D.** Hemophilia is a congenital bleeding disorder that will affect the patient during surgery; hemophilia is a clotting deficiency.

83. **A.** To avoid complications including cardiovascular and respiratory complications, the OR table is slowly leveled.

84. **C.** The vagus (X) is the cranial nerve that innervates the pharynx, larynx, external auditory meatus and thoracic and abdominal muscles.

85. **D.** Cefazolin sodium is in the class of cephalosporin antibiotics.

86. **D.** Atropine sulfate is a common mydriatic drug.

87. **D.** Bolsters are used with retention sutures to prevent the suture from cutting into the skin surface.

88. **B.** Pulse oximetry is a noninvasive method of measuring the blood oxygenation.

89. **C.** The parietal bones form the greater portion of the sides and roof of the cranial cavity.

90. **B.** Ketamine is a dissociative agent that produces amnesia and profound analgesia; it is administered IM or IV and due to its disadvantages is limited to use on children 2-10 years old.

91. **A.** Epidural anesthesia is often used in obstetrics to produce painless child birth; it is replacing caudal anesthesia.

92. **C.** The meter is the basic unit of length in the metric system.

93. **D.** Phagocytosis is a cells ability to engulf a solid particle and digest it; it is an important defense in helping the body fight disease.

94. **A.** The hypoglossal (XII) cranial nerve carries motor fibers to the tongue and sensory impulses from the tongue to the brain.

95. **A.** Osteoarthritis is a degenerative joint disease that occurs with age; the articular cartilage is worn and the two bones move against each other causing pain due to the friction.

96. **D.** There are three types of hydrocephalus: noncommunicating, communicating, and improper absorption of CSF by the arachnoid villi.

97. **D.** Some bacterial species are capable of spore formation in order to survive harsh environmental conditions; spores are difficult to destroy.

98. **C.** The anterior and lateral walls of the trachea are supported by 15-20 C-shaped hyaline cartilage to keep the trachea from collapsing.

99. **D.** The thrombin used in the OR is of bovine origin; thrombin is a part of the blood-clotting mechanism.

100. **B.** The appendicular skeleton consists of the shoulders, arms, pelvis and legs.

101. **C.** The rate of absorption depends on many factors including type of drug preparation, dosage, route of administration and patient's health condition.

102. **C.** A Colles fracture is an angulated fracture of the distal radius located at the epiphysis about 1 in. from the wrist joint.

103. **A.** The olfactory (I) cranial nerve carries impulses for the sense of smell.

104. **C.** The purpose of the surgical hand scrub is to reduce the microbial count and render them surgically clean.

105. **C.** The extremity or end of a bone is the epiphysis.

106. **D.** The combining form that means kidney is ren/o such as renal.

107. **A.** The wisp-like nerve roots at the end of the spinal cord are called cauda equina.

108. **A.** Pneumatic tourniquet is an external mechanical method of hemostasis.

109. **B.** An aneurysm is a weak sac formed by the dilatation of the arterial walls.

110. **B.** Some bacterial species are capable of spore formation in order to survive harsh environmental conditions; spores are difficult to destroy.

111. **C.** The suffix –rrhea means discharge or flow such as menorrhea.

112. **D.** The tympanic cavity located in the middle ear contains the malleus, incus and stapes.

113. **A.** Miotics constrict the pupil by acting on the sphincter of the iris; one miotic drug is pilocarpine hydrochloride.

114. **C.** Afferent neurons, also called sensory neurons, carry nerve impulses to the CNS.

115. **C.** A differential count determines the distribution of the different kinds of WBCs through counting and providing a percentage of the total examined in the stained blood smear.

116. **C.** Chromic suture is treated with a salt solution to decrease its absorbability.

117. **B.** Scoliosis is recognized by a lateral curvature of the spinal column, deformity of the rib cage and vertebrae.

118. **D.** Sterile bottles of fluid should never be recapped; replacing the cap contaminates the inner fluid.

119. **A.** Binary fission is the simple division that results in two cells; most bacteria divide by binary fission.

120. **A.** The dome-shaped portion of the uterus located above the uterine tubes is the fundus.

121. **B.** Warfarin is an anticoagulant that prohibits the action of vitamin K.

122. **D.** Neostigmine bromide (Prostigmin) is a neuromuscular blocker.

123. **B.** Eucaryote's cellular structure is complex and procaryotes is simple with no membrane to contain the organelles.

124. **B.** The innermost thin layer of endothelium is the endocardium.

125. **C.** The normal WBC is 5,000-10,000; above that means an infection could be present.

126. **D.** The function of hemoglobin is to carry oxygen.

127. **A.** The ECG is a noninvasive method used to monitor the rate, rhythm and contractions of the heart; used to detect dysrhythmias.

128. **A.** The primary source of airborne bacteria in the O.R. is the surgical team that shed microbes from their skin.

129. **C.** The parotid is one of three pairs of salivary glands; it is located anterior and inferior to the ears.

130. **B.** HIV, human immunodeficiency virus, is the cause of Acquired Immunodeficiency Syndrome.

131. **D.** Stapling devices do not retract.

132. **B.** The acromion is part of the scapula or shoulder blade.

133. **B.** Evisceration is the rupture of a wound with the spilling of contents.

134. **C.** The knee joint is cushioned by the lateral and medial meniscus that are situated on the upper articular surface of the tibia.

135. **C.** The axillary region should be considered non-sterile once the gown has been donned.

136. **D.** One meter equals 1,000 millimeters.

137. **C.** The calcaneus is one of seven tarsal bones; it is the largest of the tarsal bones located inferiorly to the talus and forms the heel.

138. **C.** The diaphysis is the shaft, or long, main part of the bone.

139. **C.** Viruses that invade bacteria are called bacteriophages.

140. **B.** Another name for spongy bone is cancellous.

141. **A.** 8-0 suture size is used for microvascular and eye procedures.

142. **D.** There are 12 pairs of ribs; the first 7 pairs are called the true ribs that join anteriorly with the sternum by costal cartilages.

143. **C.** The suffix –trophy means development or nourishment such as hypertrophy.

144. **B.** Second intention (granulation) healing occurs in large wounds that cannot be approximated due to loss of tissue or an infection has caused tissue necrosis.

145. **D.** Class IV Dirty/Infected has the highest rate of wound infection since it is an open traumatic wound, preoperative microbial contamination or perforated viscus.

146. **D.** Atrophy refers to wasting or decrease in size of a body part due to disease or other reasons such as muscle atrophy due to lack of exercise.

147. **B.** *C. perfringens* is the microbe that is responsible for causing gas gangrene, a serious type of deep wound infection.

148. **A.** Furosemide is a diuretic used to maintain intraoperative urinary output.

149. **D.** Stainless steel suture has high tensile strength and can support a wound indefinitely.

150. **D.** Lasix is a diuretic that prevents reabsorption of sodium and water in the kidney; it is given intraoperatively to maintain urinary output.

151. **A.** Cilia and flagella are two methods by which bacteria can achieve motility.

152. **B.** Drugs can cause undesirable effects such as diarrhea, dizziness, drowsiness and constipation, but do not cause hemorrhage.

153. **C.** Emergence occurs at the end of the surgical procedure with the goal of having the patient as awake as possible by the end of the procedure.

154. **C.** Suture ligature is another name for stick tie.

155. **D.** Oxytocin is an oxytocic drug that is used to induce or continue labor and contract the uterus following delivery to control hemorrhage.

156. **D.** Finger-like projections located on the end of the fallopian tube are the fimbriae.

157. **A.** The six rights are right patient, right drug, right dose, right route of administration, right time and frequency, right documentation and labeling.

158. **C.** The prostate is a gland that is conical shaped that lies under the bladder and the urethra travels through it.

159. **D.** Agar is an agent added to a growth medium to solidify the medium.

160. **B.** Vicryl™ is another name for polyglactin 910, which is the synthetic chemical used to make the suture material.

161. **C.** The prefix epi- means above and upon such as epicondyle.

162. **C.** Tendons are located at the end of muscles and attaches the muscle to bone; ligaments attach bone to bone.

163. **D.** The sections of the stomach are the upper fundus, cardia, corpus, antrum and pylorus.

164. **C.** A needle with a cutting point is used on tendon.

165. **C.** The left coronary artery divides into the anterior interventricular and circumflex.

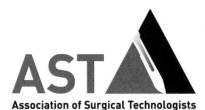

ASSOCIATION OF SURGICAL TECHNOLOGISTS

BONUS SCIENCE REVIEW QUESTIONS #2

1. **Where does the exchange of gases take place in the lung?**

    o   A.   Bronchi

    o   B.   Trachea

    o   C.   Alveoli

    o   D.   Larynx

2. **One of the distinguishing features of viruses is that they are:**

    o   A.   Saprophytic hosts

    o   B.   Obligate intracellular parasites

    o   C.   Nonpathogenic microorganisms

    o   D.   Gram-positive microorganisms

3. **Which of the following would have a positive effect on wound healing?**

    o   A.   Radiation therapy

    o   B.   Use of steroids

    o   C.   Deficiency in vitamin K

    o   D.   Early ambulation

4. **Which of the following is a hypertrophic scar formation?**

    o   A.   Keloid

    o   B.   Granulation

    o   C.   Dead space

    o   D.   Cicatrix

5. **Where is cerebrospinal fluid formed?**

   o A. Auricles

   o B. Superior sagittal sinus

   o C. Cerebellum

   o D. Choroid plexuses

6. **Which of the following arteries supplies blood to the brain?**

   o A. Carotid

   o B. Brachial

   o C. Aorta

   o D. Femoral

7. **The preoperative medication used to neutralize stomach acidity is:**

   o A. Diazepam (Valium®)

   o B. Propofol (Diprivan®)

   o C. Epinephrine (Adrenalin®)

   o D. Sodium citrate (Bi-Citra®)

8. **Which of the following are procaryotic?**

   o A. Plants

   o B. Molds

   o C. Bacteria

   o D. Protozoa

9. **Which of the following is a passive drain that allows fluid to exit by capillary action?**

   o A. T-tube

   o B. Penrose

   o C. Hemovac

   o D. Jackson-Pratt

10. **The colon ends at the:**

    o A. Anal canal

    o B. Ascending colon

    o C. Ileocecal valve

    o D. Cecum and transverse colon

11. **Which of the following is a narcotic antagonist?**

    o A. Protamine sulfate

    o B. Naloxone hydrochloride (Narcan®)

    o C. Vecuronium (Norcuron®)

    o D. Diazepam (Valium®)

12. **The combining form meaning gland is:**

o A. Myom/o

o B. Aden/o

o C. Sarc/o

o D. Arthro/o

13. **Which of the following ligaments suspends the uterus?**

o A. Falciform

o B. Cruciate

o C. Treitz

o D. Broad

14. **What type of scar formation is considered hypertrophic?**

o A. Keloid

o B. Cicatrix

o C. Dermoid

o D. Adhesion

15. **Diuretics are used intraoperatively to:**

o A. Increase blood volume

o B. Decrease urine output

o C. Decrease intracranial pressure

o D. Increase clotting time

16. **The type of surgical laser is determined by its:**

o A. Active medium

o B. Resonator cavity

o C. Semi-conductor

o D. Pump source

17. **What does the prefix "contra-" mean?**

o A. Against, opposite

o B. Down, inferior

o C. Thorough, complete

o D. Difficult, abnormal

18. **The brain contains how many ventricles?**

o A. 2

o B. 3

o C. 4

o D. 5

19. **The anatomical structure that creates cerebrospinal fluid is the:**

    o A. Pineal gland
    o B. Pons
    o C. Choroid plexuses
    o D. Aqueduct of Sylvius

20. **Which salivary gland is drained by Stensen's duct?**

    o A. Sublingual
    o B. Tonsilar
    o C. Parotid
    o D. Submandibular

21. **The type of fracture that is caused by forcing one bone upon another is called:**

    o A. Oblique
    o B. Greenstick
    o C. Simple
    o D. Impacted

22. **Irregular shaped bones that develop in the sutures of the skull are called:**

    o A. Flat
    o B. Wormian
    o C. Vomer
    o D. Sesamoid

23. **Which term refers to the end of a bone?**

    o A. Epiphysis
    o B. Trochanter
    o C. Condyle
    o D. Diaphysis

24. **Which of the following is the most inert in tissue?**

    o A. Polypropylene
    o B. Nylon
    o C. Polyster
    o D. Chromic

25. **Immediately after receiving a medication, the surgical technologist in the scrub role should:**

    o A. Label the medication
    o B. Administer the medication
    o C. Measure and fill the syringe
    o D. Cover the medication cup to avoid contamination

26. **What classification is a Bake surgical instrument?**

  o A. Clamping
  o B. Dilating
  o C. Grasping
  o D. Cutting

27. **The wavelength of laser light:**

  o A. Is never visible
  o B. Ranges from infrared to deep ultraviolet
  o C. Is always visible
  o D. Ranges red to violet

28. **Which laser should not be used in the presence of clear fluids?**

  o A. Holmium: YAG
  o B. Nd:YAG
  o C. Argon
  o D. Carbon dioxide

29. **The abnormal enlargement of the male breast is called:**

  o A. Gynecomastia
  o B. Mammoplasty
  o C. Adenopathy
  o D. Mastodynia

30. **What is the classification of Surgilon™?**

  o A. Synthetic absorbable monofilament
  o B. Synthetic nonabsorbable multifilament
  o C. Natural absorbable monofilament
  o D. Natural nonabsorbable multifiliment

31. **The inferior portion of the brain stem is the:**

  o A. Midbrain
  o B. Medulla
  o C. Hypothalamus
  o D. Pons

32. **In which surgical procedure would blunt needles be used?**

  o A. Face lift
  o B. Eye enucleation
  o C. Valve replacement
  o D. Liver resection

33. **The second cervical vertebra is called the:**

- o A. Lamina
- o B. Atlas
- o C. Axis
- o D. Body

34. **The largest ball-and-socket joint is the:**

- o A. Hip
- o B. Shoulder
- o C. Elbow
- o D. Knee

35. **What does the suffix -otomy mean?**

- o A. Protrusion
- o B. Excision
- o C. Incision
- o D. Fusion

36. **The inner most layer of the eye is called the:**

- o A. Choroid
- o B. Retina
- o C. Cornea
- o D. Sclera

37. **The colon begins at the:**

- o A. Cecum
- o B. Jejunum
- o C. Ileum
- o D. Sigmoid

38. **Which of the following makes up the inner tunic of the eye and receives images?**

- o A. Retina
- o B. Rods
- o C. Cones
- o D. Ciliary body

39. **An example of a flat bone is the:**

- o A. Zygoma
- o B. Cranial
- o C. Calcaneous
- o D. Vertebra

40. **Laser light travels:**

o A. According to the Earth's curvature
o B. In a straight line
o C. In an arc
o D. According to the pull of gravity

41. **What is the primary function of the islets of Langerhans?**

o A. Breakdown of fat
o B. Maintain blood sugar level
o C. Maintain urinary glucose level
o D. Increase oxygen level in blood

42. **1cc of solution is equivalent to:**

o A. 1L
o B. 1mL
o C. 100mL
o D. 10mL

43. **What does the abbreviation NPO mean?**

o A. No liquids
o B. Only clear liquids
o C. No food after midnight
o D. Nothing by mouth

44. **The prefix "hemi-" means:**

o A. Beneath
o B. Between
o C. Not
o D. Half

45. **A solid granular mass that develops on the ovary after the release of an ovum is the:**

o A. Graafian follicle
o B. Stroma
o C. Corpus luteum
o D. Zygote

46. **Muscle is attached to bone by:**

o A. Fascia
o B. Tendon
o C. Ligament
o D. Cartilage

47. **Which of the following is a monofilament nonabsorbable suture?**

    o A. Nurolon™

    o B. Ethibond™

    o C. Prolene™

    o D. Monocryl™

48. **The abnormal congenital opening of the male urethra on the underside of the penis is referred to as:**

    o A. Hypospadias

    o B. Epispadias

    o C. Cystocele

    o D. Phimosis

49. **All of the medications inhibit blood coagulation, except:**

    o A. Warfarin

    o B. Calcium

    o C. Heparin

    o D. Aspirin

50. **A patient with indirect and direct hernia has what type of hernia?**

    o A. Pantaloon

    o B. Sliding

    o C. Ventral

    o D. Femoral

51. **What degrees is 98.6 Farenheit equal to in Celsius?**

    o A. 35

    o B. 36

    o C. 37

    o D. 38

52. **Which of the following is a large vein that drains the head?**

    o A. Saphenous

    o B. Jugular

    o C. Subclavian

    o D. Brachial

53. **The smallest microorganisms known are:**

    o A. Rickettsias

    o B. Bacteria

    o C. Viruses

    o D. Protozoa

54. **Which of the following is the outer layer of the colon?**

o A. Serosa

o B. Submucosa

o C. Muscularis

o D. Mucosa

55. **Which of the following structures are found in the ventricles of the heart?**

o A. Papillary muscles

o B. Ligamentum arteriosum

o C. Pectinate muscles

o D. Fossa ovalis

56. **Microfibrillar collagen (Avitene®) is a/an:**

o A. Antibiotic

o B. CNS depressant

o C. Hemostatic agent

o D. Steroid hormone

57. **A curved, tapered surgical needle is used most often on what type of tissue?**

o A. Intestine

o B. Skin

o C. Tendon

o D. Eye

58. **What is the pharmacological action of hydrocortisone?**

o A. Miotic

o B. Sedative

o C. Anti-histamine

o D. Anti-inflammatory

59. **The passage of fluid and dissolved material into the thin membrane of a cell wall is:**

o A. Commensalism

o B. Diffusion

o C. Symbiosis

o D. Osmosis

60. **The suffix that refers to suturing is:**

o A. -rrhagia

o B. -rrhea

o C. -rrhaphy

o D. -tomy

61. **Which combining form means eyelid?**

o A. Ophthalm/o

o B. Dacry/o

o C. Blephar/o

o D. Ot/o

62. **Inflammation of the inner lining of the heart caused by bacteria is known as:**

o A. Chondritis

o B. Endocarditis

o C. Gastritis

o D. Pericarditis

63. **What portion of the back table is considered sterile once the sterile field has been established?**

o A. Top of the table to within 1" of edge of the drape

o B. Up to 2 inches below table level

o C. Only the top

o D. Entire length, width and sides of the table

64. **Which laser beam can travel through clear tissues without heating them?**

o A. Neodymium: YAG

o B. Carbon dioxide

o C. Argon

o D. Excimer

65. **The thyroid gland consists of right and left lobes joined by the:**

o A. Corpus callosum

o B. Larynx

o C. Isthmus

o D. Cricoid cartilage

66. **The use of silk suture in urinary or biliary tract may result in:**

o A. Emboli

o B. Stricture

o C. Dehiscence

o D. Calculi

67. **Which nerve is affected by carpal tunnel syndrome?**

o A. Ulnar

o B. Median

o C. Radial

o D. Brachial

68. **Which division of the nervous system controls involuntary muscle contractions?**

o A. Afferent

o B. Central

o C. Somatic

o D. Autonomic

69. **Which of the following glands regulates body temperature?**

o A. Thalamus

o B. Adrenal

o C. Pituitary

o D. Hypothalamus

70. **Which two drug classifications are combined to produce neuroleptanalgesia?**

o A. Tranquilizer and narcotic

o B. Cholinergic and antimuscarinic

o C. Anti-histamine and sedative

o D. Adrenergic and diuretic

71. **Removal of necrotic tissue is called:**

o A. Debridement

o B. Excoriation

o C. Z-plasty

o D. Dermabrasion

72. **Cramplike pains in the lower leg caused by poor blood circulation to the lower leg muscles is called:**

o A. Claudication

o B. Embolism

o C. Ischemia

o D. Thrombosis

73. **The gram stain differentiates between:**

o A. Living and dead organisms

o B. Fungi

o C. Bacteria

o D. Viruses and bacteria

74. **When opening an envelope-folded wrapper containing a sterile item the first flap is opened:**

o A. According to preference

o B. Away from self

o C. Toward self

o D. To the side

75. **Which nasal sinus is entered through an eyebrow incision?**

o A. Sphenoid

o B. Ethmoid

o C. Frontal

o D. Maxillary

76. **Craniosynostosis is a/an:**

o A. Premature closure of cranial sutures

o B. Infection of the subdural space

o C. Improper absorption of CSF

o D. Congenital collection of abnormal vessels

77. **Which of the following joints permits movement in only one plane?**

o A. Condyloid

o B. Saddle

o C. Hinge

o D. Gliding

78. **Hepatomegaly is:**

o A. Enlarged liver

o B. Small kidney

o C. Cancer of the liver

o D. Enlarged spleen

79. **What is the general rule for prepping a contaminated area?**

o A. Prep the surrounding area last and the contaminated area first, using a separate sponge

o B. No special considerations are necessary

o C. Prep the surrounding area first and the contaminated area last, using a separate sponge

o D. Contaminated areas need not be prepped

80. **The kneecap is also known as the:**

o A. Patella

o B. Tibia

o C. Popliteal

o D. Fibula

81. **Topical administration of drugs includes all the following, except:**

o A. Sublingual

o B. Transdermal

o C. Buccal

o D. Parenteral

82. **Which quadrant is the appendix located?**

o A. Left upper
o B. Right upper
o C. Right lower
o D. Left lower

83. **Albumin, globulin, and fibrinogen are:**

o A. Formed elements of blood
o B. Coagulation factors
o C. Plasma proteins
o D. Hematopoietic growth factors

84. **A projection on the surface of a bone located above a condyle is called a:**

o A. Tubercle
o B. Medial condyle
o C. Tuberosity
o D. Epicondyle

85. **The peripheral nervous system contains:**

o A. Spinal cord and spinal nerves
o B. Cranial and spinal nerves
o C. Cranial nerves and spinal cord
o D. Brain and spinal cord

86. **The olecranon process is part of which bone?**

o A. Ulna
o B. Scapula
o C. Radius
o D. Humerus

87. **The vertebrae are examples of what type of bone?**

o A. Long
o B. Irregular
o C. Flat
o D. Short

88. **Which of the following medical terms refers to the skin?**

o A. Digestive
o B. Endocrine
o C. Integumentary
o D. Respiratory

89.   **Retinal detachment is due to:**

o   A.   Fibrovascular growth of conjunctiva

o   B.   Leakage of liquid from vitreous cavity

o   C.   Excessive scar tissue

o   D.   Obstruction of the nasolacrimal duct

90.   **Softening of the bone is called:**

o   A.   Osteomalacia

o   B.   Osteopenia

o   C.   Osteoarthritis

o   D.   Osteomyelitis

91.   **Which of the following refers to the ability of the body to maintain a normal internal environment?**

o   A.   Metabolism

o   B.   Homeostasis

o   C.   Syncope

o   D.   Glycolysis

92.   **Which of the following is used to perform Schiller's test?**

o   A.   Lugol's solution

o   B.   Methylene blue

o   C.   Acetic acid

o   D.   Indigo carmine

93.   **The roof of the mouth is called the:**

o   A.   Alveolus

o   B.   Palate

o   C.   Uvula

o   D.   Oropharynx

94.   **Which chemical hemostatic agent must never be injected?**

o   A.   Heparin

o   B.   Papaverine

o   C.   Thrombin

o   D.   Epinephrine

95.   **What pathological term refers to failure of the lower esophageal muscles to relax?**

o   A.   Reflux

o   B.   Diverticula

o   C.   Achalasia

o   D.   Varices

96. **What does the suffix "-stasis" mean?**

   o A. Hardening

   o B. Stopping, standing still

   o C. Drooping, prolapse

   o D. Treatment

97. **Which of the following terms refers to the level of honesty and integrity that every surgical technologist must uphold in the delivery of quality patient care?**

   o A. Primum non nocere

   o B. Sterile technique

   o C. Respondeat superior

   o D. Surgical conscience

98. **The mucous membrane covering the eye is called the:**

   o A. Choroid

   o B. Retina

   o C. Sclera

   o D. Conjunctiva

99. **The small intestine begins at the:**

   o A. Stomach

   o B. Hepatic artery

   o C. Pylorus

   o D. Ileocecal valve

100. **What clotting factor does fibrinogen react with to form fibrin during the clotting process?**

   o A. Plasma

   o B. Thrombin

   o C. Collagen

   o D. Serotonin

101. **Streptokinase is used as a/an:**

   o A. Antibiotic

   o B. Coagulant

   o C. Anticoagulant

   o D. Fibrinolytic

102. **Which of the following are eucaryotic?**

   o A. Fungi

   o B. Cyanobacteria

   o C. Bacteria

   o D. Viruses

103. **Which term refers to low blood volume?**

o A. Hypovolemia

o B. Hypokalemia

o C. Hypothermia

o D. Hypoglycemia

104. **Turning the hand so that the palm is upward is referred to as:**

o A. Pronation

o B. Supination

o C. Rotation

o D. Inversion

105. **The foramen magnum is an opening in which bone?**

o A. Occipital

o B. Parietal

o C. Sphenoid

o D. Temporal

106. **The number of pairs of cranial nerves is:**

o A. 9

o B. 10

o C. 11

o D. 12

107. **Intestinal motility is called:**

o A. Peristalsis

o B. Digestion

o C. Enteritis

o D. Stasis

108. **Healthcare associated infections refers to:**

o A. Infections in the nasal cavity

o B. Infections acquired at home

o C. Hospital acquired infections

o D. An invasion of pathogenic microorganisms

109. **Which of these local anesthetics is long acting?**

o A. Cocaine

o B. Novacaine

o C. Marcaine

o D. Xylocaine

110. **Spherically-shaped bacteria that occur in chains are referred to as:**

- o A. Diplococci
- o B. Coccobacilli
- o C. Staphylococci
- o D. Streptococci

111. **Cephalosporins are a/an:**

- o A. Antibiotic
- o B. CNS depressant
- o C. Mydriatic
- o D. Steroid

112. **Which of the following diseases is the result of invasion by a pathogen?**

- o A. Scurvy
- o B. Diabetes
- o C. Pneumonia
- o D. Rickets

113. **Atheroma within the lumen of an artery is called:**

- o A. Truncus arteriosus
- o B. Aneurysm
- o C. Arteriosclerosis obliterans
- o D. Cardiomyopathy

114. **What type of suture is used for tendon repair?**

- o A. Polydioxanone
- o B. Polyglactin 910
- o C. Polyethylene
- o D. Poliglecaprone 25

115. **Which of the following is a type of inflammatory bowel disease with chronic inflammation of the intestine?**

- o A. Pilonidal
- o B. Crohn's
- o C. Mesenteric
- o D. Diverticular

116. **What does the number 4 represent in the decimal 0.02457?**

- o A. Tenths
- o B. Hundreths
- o C. Thousandths
- o D. Ten-thousandths

117. **Stat means:**

o A. Delayed

o B. As necessary

o C. As directed

o D. Immediately

118. **What is the outermost layer of the skin?**

o A. Adipose

o B. Dermis

o C. Epidermis

o D. Subcutaneous

119. **Which syringe is the most appropriate for administering a local anesthetic?**

o A. Bulb

o B. Toomey

o C. Asepto

o D. Luer-Lok

120. **The bone that articulates with the distal tibia and fibula is the:**

o A. Talus

o B. Femur

o C. Patella

o D. Calcaneus

121. **Which directional term refers to the middle of the body?**

o A. Lateral

o B. Medial

o C. Caudal

o D. Proximal

122. **What is the correct order of the layers of the meninges anterior to posterior?**

o A. Dura, arachnoid, pia

o B. Pia, arachnoid, dura

o C. Arachnoid, dura, pia

o D. Dura, pia, arachnoid

123. **The structure connecting the spinal cord with the brain is the:**

o A. Hypothalamus

o B. Diencephalon

o C. Cerebellum

o D. Brain stem

124. **The invasion of pathogens within the tissues of a host is called:**

   o   A.   Infestation
   o   B.   Infection
   o   C.   Intussusception
   o   D.   Inflammation

125. **Reduced blood flow to an area is:**

   o   A.   Hemostasis
   o   B.   Extravasation
   o   C.   Ischemia
   o   D.   Hemorrhage

126. **The fraction 1/4 is equal to:**

   o   A.   0.25
   o   B.   0.5
   o   C.   0.75
   o   D.   1

127. **Which non-absorbable suture may be used in the presence of infection?**

   o   A.   Polypropylene
   o   B.   Plain gut
   o   C.   Silk
   o   D.   Polyglactic acid

128. **The presence of pathogenic microorganisms in the blood or tissues is called:**

   o   A.   Necrosis
   o   B.   Toxicity
   o   C.   Abscess
   o   D.   Sepsis

129. **Endorphins, enkephalins, dopamine, and serotonin are examples of:**

   o   A.   Electrolytes
   o   B.   Catecholamines
   o   C.   Hormones
   o   D.   Neurotransmitters

130. **What cellular organelle serves as the site of protein synthesis?**

   o   A.   Vacuoles
   o   B.   Lysosomes
   o   C.   Ribosomes
   o   D.   Mitochondria

131. **Microorganisms that grow best with a low level of oxygen supply are:**

o A. Facultative

o B. Microaerophiles

o C. Aerotolerant anaerobes

o D. Spores

132. **The number of extrinsic ocular muscles that control eye movement is:**

o A. 2

o B. 4

o C. 6

o D. 8

133. **The cranial nerve that may be injured during carotid endarterectomy is the:**

o A. Facial (VII)

o B. Vagus (X)

o C. Spinal accessory (XI)

o D. Hypoglossal (XII)

134. **The term staphylococcus is the arrangement of:**

o A. Cocci in chains

o B. Bacilli in clusters

o C. Bacilli in chains

o D. Cocci in cluster

135. **Viruses reproduce by:**

o A. Mitosis

o B. Host cell metabolism

o C. Binary fission

o D. Meiosis

136. **A clinical symptom of shock is:**

o A. Hypervolemia

o B. Hypoventilation

o C. Hyperthermia

o D. Hypotension

137. **The normal pouches of the large intestine are called:**

o A. Taniae coli

o B. Haustra

o C. Polyps

o D. Diverticula

138. **Which of the following bacteria requires oxygen?**

   o A. Gram positive
   o B. Aerobic
   o C. Anaerobic
   o D. Gram negative

139. **What is the function of the Bartholin's glands?**

   o A. Produce oocytes
   o B. Secrete lubrication
   o C. Stimulate ovulation
   o D. Secrete hormones

140. **Which of the following absorbable sutures offers the longest duration of wound support?**

   o A. Polyglactin 910
   o B. Polydioxanone
   o C. Polyglyconate
   o D. Poliglecaprone 25

141. **Any instance in which a local anesthetic is injected to block or anesthetize a nerve is called:**

   o A. General anesthesia
   o B. Monitored anesthesia care
   o C. Regional anesthesia
   o D. Topical anesthesia

142. **The body's first line of defense against the invasion of pathogens is:**

   o A. Unbroken skin
   o B. Immune response
   o C. Phagocytosis
   o D. Cellular response

143. **Anticoagulants:**

   o A. Increase the clotting time
   o B. Decrease blood pressure
   o C. Decrease the clotting time
   o D. Increase blood pressure

144. **A method of anesthesia in which anesthetic medication is injected into the subarachnoid space is a/an:**

   o A. Bier block
   o B. Spinal block
   o C. Nerve block
   o D. Field block

145. **Microorganisms that have the ability to adapt to an aerobic or anaerobic environment are:**

o   A.   Aerobes
o   B.   Parasites
o   C.   Facultative
o   D.   Anaerobes

146. **Bone grafts are usually taken from the:**

o   A.   Ilium
o   B.   Ischium
o   C.   Iliac crest
o   D.   Sacrum

147. **The fifth cranial nerve is also called the:**

o   A.   Trigeminal
o   B.   Vagus
o   C.   Vestibulocochlear
o   D.   Trochlear

148. **The outer covering of the heart is called the:**

o   A.   Epicardium
o   B.   Myocardium
o   C.   Pericardium
o   D.   Endocardium

149. **Which of the following is the most common cause of a surgical site infection?**

o   A.   Incorrect surgical prep
o   B.   Improper sterilization process
o   C.   Hole in the surgeon's glove
o   D.   Patient's endogenous flora

150. **Which of the following is the staining characteristic of gram-negative organisms?**

o   A.   Stain colorless
o   B.   Stain red
o   C.   Do not consistently stain
o   D.   Stain purple

151. **The diencephalon is composed of the:**

o   A.   Thalamus and hypothalamus
o   B.   Medulla and spinal cord
o   C.   Midbrain and thalamus
o   D.   Pons and midbrain

152. **Narcotic analgesics produce their effects by:**

   o   A.   Decreasing salivation
   o   B.   Stimulating the central nervous system
   o   C.   Minimizing pain perception
   o   D.   Increasing general anesthesia required

153. **Which of the following is a life-threatening allergic reaction?**

   o   A.   Toxic shock
   o   B.   Anaphylaxis
   o   C.   Urticaria
   o   D.   Tachyphylaxis

154. **Before donning the sterile gown and gloves the surgical technologist must:**

   o   A.   Sterilize the hands
   o   B.   Perform a surgical hand and arm scrub
   o   C.   Disinfect the hands and arms
   o   D.   Remove all resident flora from hands and arms

155. **Which of the following can be achieved with the use of electrocautery?**

   o   A.   Coagulation
   o   B.   Ablation
   o   C.   Dessication
   o   D.   Fulguration

156. **Antibiotics given to prevent postoperative infection are considered:**

   o   A.   Curative
   o   B.   Palliative
   o   C.   Prophylactic
   o   D.   Maintenance

157. **The largest part of the brain is the:**

   o   A.   Thalamus
   o   B.   Hypothalamus
   o   C.   Cerebellum
   o   D.   Cerebrum

158. **The longest bone in the body is the:**

   o   A.   Femur
   o   B.   Humerus
   o   C.   Tibia
   o   D.   Pelvis

159. **What does the term hepat/o mean?**

o A. Pancreas

o B. Blood

o C. Liver

o D. Iron

160. **The folds of the lining in the stomach are:**

o A. Plicae circulares

o B. Microvilli

o C. Cristae

o D. Rugae

161. **The function of the sphincter of Oddi is to control the flow of:**

o A. CSF into the spinal cord

o B. Acids in the stomach

o C. Bile into the duodenum

o D. Urine into the bladder

162. **Heparin is measured in:**

o A. Units

o B. Cubic centimeters

o C. Milliliters

o D. Micrograms

163. **Which agent is used to perform a chromotubation?**

o A. Barium sulfate

o B. Indigo carmine

o C. Gentian violet

o D. Methylene blue

164. **The purpose of the Foley catheter is to:**

o A. Drain the bladder in order to avoid injury

o B. Secure vaginal packing postoperatively

o C. Estimate the patient's bladder capacity

o D. Verify the position of the uterers

165. **The only non-articulating bone in the body is the:**

o A. Mastoid

o B. Vomer

o C. Sphenoid

o D. Hyoid

166. **Millimeter (mm) is a unit used to measure:**

o A. Length
o B. Weight
o C. Time
o D. Volume

167. **What does the prefix inter- mean?**

o A. Within
o B. Between
o C. Below
o D. Above

168. **What is known as the measure of force required to break a suture?**

o A. Gauge
o B. Yield power
o C. Pliability
o D. Tensile strength

169. **The first cervical vertebra is called the:**

o A. Pedicle
o B. Axis
o C. Atlas
o D. Foramina

170. **The suffix meaning blood condition is:**

o A. -emia
o B. -osis
o C. -oma
o D. -ectomy

171. **What organ of the body contains both striated and smooth muscle?**

o A. Liver
o B. Heart
o C. Kidney
o D. Colon

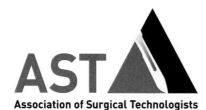
#	Ans		#	Ans		#	Ans		#	Ans		#	Ans		#	Ans
1	C		31	B		61	C		91	B		121	B		151	A
2	B		32	D		62	B		92	A		122	A		152	C
3	D		33	C		63	C		93	B		123	D		153	B
4	A		34	A		64	C		94	C		124	B		154	B
5	D		35	C		65	C		95	C		125	C		155	A
6	A		36	B		66	D		96	B		126	A		156	C
7	D		37	A		67	B		97	D		127	A		157	D
8	C		38	A		68	D		98	D		128	D		158	A
9	B		39	B		69	D		99	C		129	D		159	C
10	A		40	B		70	A		100	B		130	C		160	D
11	B		41	B		71	A		101	D		131	B		161	C
12	B		42	B		72	A		102	A		132	C		162	A
13	D		43	D		73	C		103	A		133	D		163	D
14	A		44	D		74	B		104	B		134	D		164	A
15	C		45	C		75	C		105	A		135	B		165	D
16	A		46	B		76	A		106	D		136	D		166	A
17	A		47	C		77	C		107	A		137	B		167	B
18	C		48	A		78	A		108	C		138	B		168	D
19	C		49	B		79	A		109	C		139	B		169	C
20	C		50	A		80	A		110	D		140	B		170	A
21	D		51	C		81	D		111	A		141	C		171	B
22	B		52	B		82	C		112	C		142	A			
23	A		53	C		83	C		113	C		143	C			
24	A		54	A		84	D		114	C		144	B			
25	A		55	A		85	B		115	B		145	C			
26	B		56	C		86	A		116	C		146	C			
27	B		57	A		87	B		117	D		147	A			
28	D		58	D		88	C		118	C		148	C			
29	A		59	D		89	B		119	D		149	D			
30	B		60	C		90	A		120	A		150	B			

1. **C.** Bronchioles end in the clusters of grape-like structures called the alveoli where the exchange of oxygen and carbon dioxide takes place.

2. **B.** Viruses are obligate intracellular parasites, meaning they rely completely on the host cells for survival.

3. **D.** Early ambulation is one of the most important factors in the recovery of the surgical patient; therefore, it would not interfere with the healing process for a patient.

4. **A.** Keloid scar formation is a hypertrophic scar formation that often occurs in dark-skinned individuals.

5. **D.** Cerebrospinal fluid (CSF) is formed in the choroid plexuses of the brain.

6. **A.** The internal carotid and vertebral arteries supply blood to the brain.

7. **D.** Sodium citrate is an H2 blocker that neutralizes stomach acid and is given preoperatively.

8. **C.** All bacteria are procaryotes (also spelled prokaryotes).

9. **B.** The Penrose drain is a type of passive drain; one end is inserted into the wound and the other is outside the wound to allow the fluid to move out of the wound to be absorbed by the dressing.

10. **A.** The last section of the colon is the anal canal ending in the anal orifice called the anus.

11. **B.** Naloxone hydrochloride is a narcotic antagonist used to reverse narcotic analgesics.

12. **B.** The combining form aden/o means gland such as adenoma.

13. **D.** The broad ligament is one of four ligaments that extend from the pelvic walls and suspend the uterus.

14. **A.** Hypertrophy occurs when the body over-produces collagen; therefore the scar formation would be a Keloid.

15. **C.** Diuretics such as mannitol are used to decrease ICP, IOP or edema.

16. **A.** Lasers are named according to the active medium that is used such as gas, solid, liquid or semiconductor crystals.

17. **A.** The prefix contra means against or opposite such as contralateral.

18. **C.** The lateral ventricles are located in each cerebral hemisphere; third ventricle is located between the halves of the thalamus; fourth ventricle is located in the brain stem.

19. **C.** The choroid plexuses are networks of capillaries located in the walls of the ventricles and are responsible for producing CSF.

20. **C.** The excretory duct of the parotid salivary gland is Stenson's duct.

21. **D.** An impacted fracture is when the broken ends of bones are forced into each other creating bone fragments.

22. **B.** Small, irregular shaped bones located within the sutures of cranial bones are called sutural or Wormian bones; the number of bones varies with each person.

23. **A.** The epiphyses (plural; epiphysis, sing.) are the proximal and distal ends of the bone.

24. **A.** Polypropylene is one of the most inert suture materials.

25. **A.** Immediately after a medication is transferred to the sterile field the CST must label it.

26. **B.** The Bakes common duct dilator comes in a set of sequentially sized dilators #3-#10.

27. **B.** The wavelength of laser light energy extends from near-ultraviolet to far-infrared.

28. **D.** The carbon dioxide laser beam is absorbed by water, therefore it is not effective for transmitting through clear liquids.

29. **A.** Gynecomastia refers to the excess development of the male breast due to pathological or physiological reasons.

30. **B.** Surgilon is an example of a nylon suture. It is braided nylon with minimal tissue reaction and is coated to reduce tissue drag.

31. **B.** The medulla portion of the brain is a continuation of the spinal cord and forms the inferior portion of the brain stem.

32. **D.** A blunt needle would be used for a liver resection due to the tissue being so friable.

33. **C.** Seven bones are located in the cervical region; the second cervical vertebra (C2) is the axis which is fused with the body of the atlas.

34. **A.** The hip joint is a ball-and-socket joint formed by the head of the femur that fits into the acetabulum of the pelvis.

35. **C.** Otomy means incision.

36. **B.** The third innermost layer of the eye is the retina that lines the posterior 3/4 of the eyeball.

37. **A.** The large intestine begins at the cecum; cecum begins inferior to the ileocecal valve.

38. **A.** The retina is the inner tunic that contains the photoreceptors; it receives images.

39. **B.** The cranial bones are examples of flat bones.

40. **B.** Laser light travels in a straight line called collimated.

41. **B.** The islets of Langerhans are endocrine glands that consist of alpha cells and beta cells; the main function is to maintain normal blood sugar level.

42. **B.** 1 cubic centimer is equal to 1 milliliter.

43. **D.** NPO (nil per os) stands for nothing by mouth.

44. **D.** Hemi- means half such as in hemicolectomy.

45. **C.** The corpus luteum is a granular yellow body that develops in the ovary after the extrusion of an ovum.

46. **B.** Tendons are tough connective tissue that attach the muscles to bones.

47. **C.** Polypropylene suture includes Prolene™ and Surgilene™; it is a synthetic available as a monofilament nonabsorbable.

48. **A.** Hypospadias is the abnormal urethral opening on the underside of the penis, perineum of the male or vagina of the female.

49. **B.** Calcium is used as a blood coagulating agent to promote clot formation.

50. **A.** A pantaloon hernia is the presence of a direct and indirect hernia.

51. **C.** 98.6 - 32 = 66.6; 66.6 ÷ 1.8 = 37 degrees C.

52. **B.** The jugular vein is a large vein that drains blood from the head.

53. **C.** Viruses are the smallest microbe ranging from 300 nm to 30 nm.

54. **A.** The layers of the colon from outside to inside are serosa, muscularis, submucosa, and mucosa.

55. **A.** The papillary muscles are found in the ventricles of the heart.

56. **C.** Collagen is available in various forms one of which is Avitene®; it is available in powder form, sheets and dispensor.

57. **A.** A curved, tapered needle is used most often in soft tissue such as bowel or intestine or subcutaneous tissue.

58. **D.** Hydrocortisone sodium succinate decreases inflammation by suppressing the immune response.

59. **D.** Osmosis is a type of diffusion where fluid and dissolved solvents move from an area of lower concentration to area of higher concentration.

60. **C.** The suffix rrhaphy means to suture such as herniorrhaphy.

61. **C.** Blephar/o refers to the eyelid such as blepharoplasty.

62. **B.** Endocarditis can involve the lining of the chambers of the heart, but it usually refers to inflammation of the endocardium that covers the valves.

63. **C.** Sterile drapes once positioned should not be moved, since the portion that falls below the table edge is considered contaminated. The top only of the back table is considered sterile.

64. **C.** The argon laser beam can travel through clear fluids and tissues making it the laser of choice for treating diabetic retinopathy.

65. **C.** The right and left lateral lobes of the thyroid gland are joined by tissue that lies between the lobes and anterior to the trachea called the isthmus.

66. **D.** The use of silk suture in urinary or biliary tract may result in calculi.

67. **B.** Carpal tunnel syndrome is caused by pressure of the median nerve by the transverse carpal ligament.

68. **D.** The autonomic nervous system (ANS) controls contractions of involuntary muscles.

69. **D.** Body temperature is regulated by the hypothalamus by monitoring the processes of heat production and loss.

70. **A.** Neuroleptanalgesia is achieved with a balanced combination of a tranquilizer (neuroleptic) and narcotic analgesic agent.

71. **A.** Contaminated wounds that contain infected and/or necrosed tissue may require excision of the tissue called debridement.

72. **A.** A primary sign and symptom of arterial disease is claudication, a cramping ache due to muscle ischemia.

73. **C.** The Gram stain is used to differentiate between Gram-positive and Gram-negative bacteria.

74. **B.** The first flap is opened away from self, side flaps laterally and last flap towards self.

75. **C.** The frontal sinus is drained through an external incision made along the inferior edge of the eyebrow.

76. **A.** Craniosynostosis is the abnormal premature closure of the cranial sutures of an infant; it is treated by craniotomy.

77. **C.** The hinge joint allows movement in only one plane such as the elbow joint.

78. **A.** Hepat/o is the combining form that means liver; megaly is a suffix meaning enlarged. Therefore, hepatomegaly is the abnormal enlargment of the liver.

79. **A.** Certain areas of the body are considered contaminated; the contaminated area is prepped last and the surrounding area first using a separate sponge for both areas.

80. **A.** The patella is a small triangular-shaped sesamoid bone that rests on the anterior surface of the knee joint.

81. **D.** Topical administration includes buccal, sublingual, instillation and inhalation.

82. **C.** The appendix is located in the right lower quadrant of the abdomen.

83. **C.** Albumin, globulin, and fibrinogen are all plasma proteins.

84. **D.** An epicondyle is a projection on the surface of the bone that is located proximal to the condyle.

85. **B.** The peripheral nervous system (PNS) consists of cranial and spinal nerves.

86. **A.** The olecranon is part of the ulna.

87. **B.** Irregular bones are of a complicated shape and include such bones as the vertebrae and certain facial bones.

88. **C.** The integumentary system consists of two layers: epidermis and dermis.

89. **B.** A tear in the retina allows the liquid from the vitreous cavity to leak through the tear and collect under the retina separating it from the choroid.

90. **A.** Osteomalacia is a disease condition that causes softening of the bones caused by abnormal calcium deposits.

91. **B.** The daily actions and reactions of the body, such as maintaining the normal blood sugar level in the body, to maintain a normal physiological balance is called homeostasis.

92. **A.** Schiller's test involves applying Lugol's solution to the cervical os with a sponge stick; the tissue that remains brown colored is normal tissue and tissue that does not stain brown demonstrates dysplasia.

93. **B.** The roof of the mouth is the palate that is divided into the hard and soft palates.

94. **C.** Thrombin is used as a topical hemostatic and should never be injected.

95. **C.** Achalasia is a type of motility disorder characterized by weight loss and aspiration pneumonia.

96. **B.** The suffix stasis means standing, stopping or still such as hemostasis.

97. **D.** Surgical conscience is the basis for the practice of strict adherence to sterile technique and the ability to recognize and correct breaks in technique whether committed in the presence of others or alone.

98. **D.** The conjunctiva is the mucous membrane that lines the inner surface of the eyelid and over the sclera and cornea.

99. **C.** The small intestine begins at the pyloric sphincter located at the junction of the stomach with the duodenum.

100. **B.** Prothrombin reacts with thromboplastin to form thrombin that reacts with fibrinogen to form fibrin.

101. **D.** Streptokinase activates plasminogen to cause fibrinolysis of thrombi in treatment of MI.

102. **A.** Eucaryotes include protozoa; fungi; green, brown and red algae; and all plant and animal cells.

103. **A.** Hypovolemia refers to a low blood volume that can be the result of hemorrhage or dehydration.

104. **B.** Supination refers to pointing or turning a body part upward.

105. **A.** The foramen magnum is found in the occipital bone.

106. **D.** There are twelve pairs of cranial nerves that originate in the brain stem.

107. **A.** Peristalsis is the rhythmic contractions of the smooth muscle layer to move food forward in the intestine, urine through the ureters and bile through the CBD.

108. **C.** HAIs (formerly called nosocomial) are infections acquired in the healthcare facility as a result of healthcare intervention.

109. **C.** Marcaine is four times more potent than lidocaine and takes longer to take effect, but has a longer duration.

110. **D.** A chain of bacteria is called streptococci.

111. **A.** Cephalosporins such as Ancef®, Kefzol®, and Keflex® are antibiotics.

112. **C.** *Streptococcus pneumoniae* is the primary cause of bacterial pneumonia.

113. **C.** Arteriosclerosis obliterans affects the arterial system and is characterized by the formation of atheroma in the lumen of an artery.

114. **C.** Polyethylene is a nonabsorbable, braided suture and has a high tensile strength making it ideal for tendon repair.

115. **B.** Crohn's is an autoimmune disease that causes inflammation of the distal section of the small intestine.

116. **C.** The number 4 represents thousandths since it is three spaces after the decimal point.

117. **D.** Stat means immediately such as a stat cesarean section.

118. **C.** The integumentary system consists of the outer epidermis and inner dermis layers.

119. **D.** Luer-Lok syringes have a secure connection that locks the needle onto the syringe by twisting it on.

120. **A.** The talus is one of the seven tarsal bones that articulates with the fibula and tibia.

121. **B.** Medial means towards the middle or midline of the body; opposite is lateral.

122. **A.** The layers in order from outside to inside are dura, arachnoid and pia maters.

123. **D.** The brain stem is located between the spinal cord and diencephalon.

124. **B.** The invasion and multiplication of microbes within a host is called an infection.

125. **C.** Ischemia is the reduction of blood flow to an area.

126. **A.** $1 \div 4 = 0.25$

127. **A.** Polypropylene, besides steel, is one of the most inert suture materials that can be used in the presence of infection.

128. **D.** Sepsis refers to the presence of pathogens and/or their toxins in tissue or blood resulting in an infection.

129. **D.** Neurotransmitters are chemicals released by neurons to increase or inhibit impulses.

130. **C.** Ribosomes are an organelle composed of RNA and protein that function in the synthesis of protein.

131. **B.** Microaerophiles need oxygen, but at a lower level than what is found in room air.

132. **C.** The six extrinsic muscles of the eye originate from the bones of the orbit to move the eye in all directions.

133. **D.** The hypoglossal nerve must be identified and preserved during a carotid endarterectomy; the hypoglossal canal courses through the neck to supply the muscles of the tongue.

134. **D.** Staphylococcus refers to a cluster of bacteria.

135. **B.** Viral replication is dependent on the nucleic acid within the host cell.

136. **D.** In the adult, the clinical symptoms of shock are tachycardia, hypovolemia and hypotension.

137. **B.** The pouches of the large intestine are called haustra.

138. **B.** Aerobic bacteria require oxygen to survive; there are two types: obligate aerobes and microaerophiles.

139. **B.** Bartholin's glands are located in the vestibule; they are a pair of glands that secrete a thick lubricating mucoid fluid.

140. **B.** Polydioxanone (PDS®) is an absorbable suture that offers extended wound support.

141. **C.** Regional anesthesia is the administration of an anesthetic drug along a major nerve tract; types include Bier, spinal and epidural blocks.

142. **A.** Intact skin is the primary barrier against the invasion of pathogens.

143. **C.** Anticoagulants prevent blood clot formation and are used during vascular procedures.

144. **B.** Spinal anesthesia involves injection of an anesthetic agent into the CSF in the subarachnoid space between meningeal layers.

145. **C.** Facultative microbes can survive in an environment that contains oxygen or no oxygen.

146. **C.** The iliac crest is the best source for obtaining autogenous cancellous and cortical bone for grafting purposes.

147. **A.** The trigeminal is also called the fifth cranial nerve.

148. **C.** The pericardium protects the heart and prevents friction against the thoracic cavity.

149. **D.** The two primary sources of SSI risk to the patient are endogenous flora and resident flora of the skin.

150. **B.** Gram-negative bacteria do not retain the crystal violet and stain red from the safranin stain.

151. **A.** The thalamus and the hypothalamus comprise the diencephalon.

152. **C.** Analgesics combine with the opiate receptors in the CNS to decrease pain perception.

153. **B.** Anaphylaxis is an allergic reaction to a substance including drugs and latex.

154. **B.** Prior to donning sterile gown and gloves the surgical technologist must perform a surgical hand and arm scrub.

155. **A.** Coagulation uses electric current to close severed vessels.

156. **C.** On a routine basis antibiotics are often administered preoperatively and postoperatively to prevent an SSI referred to as surgical prophylaxis.

157. **D.** The cerebrum is the largest portion of the brain.

158. **A.** The femur is the longest, heaviest and strongest bone in the body.

159. **C.** Hepat/o refers to liver.

160. **D.** The large folds of the stomach are called rugae.

161. **C.** The sphincter of Oddi is located where the CBD and pancreatic duct join forming the ampulla of Vater; it controls the flow of bile into the duodenum.

162. **A.** Heparin sodium is measured in units; the intraoperative normal dosage is 150-300 units/kg IV.

163. **D.** In gynecology, methylene blue solution is used during a chromotubation procedure (tubal dye study) to determine the patency of the fallopian tubes.

164. **A.** The two primary purposes of the Foley catheter are measuring the urinary output and provide bladder decompression to protect the organ from injury.

165. **D.** The hyoid bone does not articulate with any other bone; it is suspended from the styloid processes of the temporal bones by ligaments and muscles.

166. **A.** Millimeter is a metric unit of length.

167. **B.** The prefix inter-means between.

168. **D.** A suture's tensile strength is the amount of weight required to break it.

169. **C.** The first cervical vertebra is called the atlas (C1) and it supports the skull.

170. **A.** The suffix that refers to a blood condition is emia such as anemia.

171. **B.** Cardiac muscle tissue is striated, but involuntary.